# Secrets to Controlling your Weight, Cravings and Mood

Understand the biochemistry of neurotransmitters and how they determine our weight and mood

Second Revision

## Maria Emmerich

Keto Adapted

ISBN  978-1456424541

Published by Maria and Craig Emmerich

# Contents

## HAPPY FATS   1

Happy Fats . . . . . . . . . . . . . . . . . . . . . . . . . . . 1
Fighting Depression with Fat, a Clean Liver, and Sleep . . . . . . . . 3
1. Dieting and Poor Food Choices: Not Enough Fat! . . . . . . . . 17
2. Gluten, Leaky Gut and Neurotransmitters . . . . . . . . . . . 18
3. Hormone Imbalances . . . . . . . . . . . . . . . . . . . . . 22
4. Prolonged Emotional or Physical Stress . . . . . . . . . . . . 24
5. Aging . . . . . . . . . . . . . . . . . . . . . . . . . . . . 24
6. Abnormal Sleep . . . . . . . . . . . . . . . . . . . . . . . 24
7. Medications . . . . . . . . . . . . . . . . . . . . . . . . . 25
8. Neurotoxins . . . . . . . . . . . . . . . . . . . . . . . . . 25
9. Genetic Predisposition . . . . . . . . . . . . . . . . . . . . 25
10. Candida or Yeast Overgrowth . . . . . . . . . . . . . . . . 26
SEROTONIN: CONTROL CRAVINGS . . . . . . . . . . . . . . 26
GABA: CONTROL EMOTIONAL EATING . . . . . . . . . . . . . 35
ACETYLCHOLINE: DECREASE FAT STORAGE . . . . . . . . . 41
DOPAMINE: INCREASE METABOLISM . . . . . . . . . . . . . 47
SLEEP . . . . . . . . . . . . . . . . . . . . . . . . . . . . 51
SUPPLEMENTING OUR BRAIN . . . . . . . . . . . . . . . . . 64
B VITAMINS: OUR STRESS VITAMINS . . . . . . . . . . . . . 71
VITAMIN D . . . . . . . . . . . . . . . . . . . . . . . . . . 73
5-HTP: Serotonin Booster . . . . . . . . . . . . . . . . . . . 77
GLUTAMINE: GABA BOOSTER . . . . . . . . . . . . . . . . . 84
PHENYLALANINE AND L-TYROSINE: DOPAMINE BOOSTER . . . . . 85
MORE ON MAGNESIUM . . . . . . . . . . . . . . . . . . . . 90
WHAT NOW? . . . . . . . . . . . . . . . . . . . . . . . . . 96

## NOTES    98

# Happy Fats

## Happy Fats

*I started yo-yo dieting and exercising when I was 8 years old even though I was a slim child with no genetic tendency towards being even slightly overweight!*

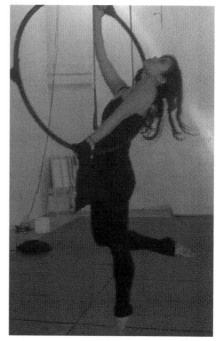

*I had started baby ballet a few months prior and was so gifted a dancer that in just a month I was moved to the advanced ballet class with the older girls and was (apparently) even better than all of them.*

*My ballet teacher who was once a prima ballerina was so impressed by my ability that she pulled my mom aside and I had the ill luck to have overheard this conversation. She told my mom that if I continued to dance that I would someday be a prima ballerina assoluta. (I had to look up this definition when I got much older but at 8 years old I had no idea what kind of compliment I was being given). But THIS I remember...she said that for me to be a ballerina I would have to go on a strict diet because I was not a 'skinny' girl. That actually my (slim) frame was not ideal for ballerinas and it would hold me back. The ballet world would think I was too 'fat' and my body was not ideal.*

*There. My life was changed at that moment. I started a lifelong struggle with body image at that moment that I heard I was too fat. And even though I stopped dancing only 2 years later, the dieting and exercise continued. I would do 45 minutes of aerobics and toning in my room with my door closed and I was only 8 years old.*

*I never had an eating disorder but I was definitely obsessed with my weight. My eating was either feast or famine because I could never stick to a real diet. I had no concept for what was healthy and what was right. I went about 'dieting very blindly. And because I could never stick to an actual 'diet' i actually started gaining weight. All the feasting was catching up to me which made me try more starvation diets only to feast later on. Because i never lost weight and I would hide my binge eating, my mom never knew how obsessed I was with my weight and my body. No one knew. It was my own secret.*

*To make a long story short, everyone in my family was thin except for me... which made me even more obsessed.*

*I have been on every diet I can think of and have been to countless nutritionists with little success. I was really at the end of the line and I always felt trapped in my body. I'm an emotional eater and have a major sweet tooth. Once I start I can't stop. I once went on a sugar binge that lasted almost a year. I felt like crap every single day!*

*Then one day, I had the good fortune to meet Maria who really understood me and my background! She showed me a lot of compassion and I knew she really cared about helping me.*

*She mapped out a great eating plan, but more importantly recommended supplements to curb my moods and emotions--which was at the crux of my emotional eating. Since then, I have bought every one of her cookbooks. I feel very educated about health and eating and can consciously make the right choices.*

*By the way, I have made almost every one of her desserts and ate it guilt free!! But I slowly stopped craving sweets altogether. When you don't deprive your body of something, it stops craving it.*

*Now, I am healthy at 5'6" and 117lbs and am no longer dieting or going crazy about my weight and body which had consumed the better part of my life. I can live and enjoy life the way I was meant to...something I haven't felt since baby ballet.*

*Thank you Maria. You are a superstar and life changer....and forever my go-to gal. I love you!*

—Romy

# Fighting Depression with Fat, a Clean Liver, and Sleep

The purpose of this chapter is to show you that uncontrollable cravings for carbohydrates that keep you from achieving keto-adaptation are not your fault. Our brain chemistry plays a huge part in how successful you will be at adapting to the keto lifestyle. So if you are plagued by depression, anxiety, or cravings, this chapter is for you!

Before I started my job as a nutritionist, Craig (my husband) and I had some really tough curve balls thrown our way. I was a rock climbing guide and I loved my job, but with the bad economy came bad news. Craig lost his job which was our main source of income. Shortly after that happened, I went to have my yearly physical and I was a puddle. I cried at the drop of a hat, worried that we were going to lose our house and our dream of adopting children. My doctor immediately thought she would be a helpful "problem-solver" by offering me an antidepressant. She did not check my vitamin D levels (which ended up being low after I had them checked with a new doctor), nor did she check my liver health, which was also probably horrible with my high-carb diet at the time. Not to mention the fact that I was also training for a marathon, which added stress to my adrenal system.

My doctor also did not ask if I took fish oil or a probiotic. All of these should be a prerequisite for patients to test and incorporate before being offered these mind-altering, addictive drugs that have lots of side effects. We would save a whole heck of a lot of money on health insurance!

On top of that she did not ask what my diet was (this is the same doctor that didn't ask about my diet when I had severe IBS — needless to say, after this visit, I changed doctors). In biology class, we are taught that our blood is manufactured and begins in the bone marrow. In Chinese medicine, we are taught that our blood begins on the end of our fork. Yep, we really are what we eat.

One of the most common and serious ailments I see in my office is depression and anxiety. Our brain and cells are over 60% fat. With the trends and tips that health magazines and commercials push on us, it is no wonder depression is sucking us all down! Before my passion for nutrition came along, I had a passion for donuts. I was an athlete and thought I could get away with eating what I wanted, as long as I worked out. Not true! Even though I ate enough calories, I was starving myself ... specifically, I was starving my brain. Even though my stomach was filled with "substance," my brain kept telling me to eat; our bodies are smart, they make us crave certain nutrients we need. In my low-fat past, I always felt guilty about enjoying fatty foods. But the human body is hard-wired to crave cholesterol and fat because our body is made up of this crucial macronutrient, so don't feel guilty! You crave cholesterol and fat because they're critical to your health. When you eat real cholesterol and fat, your body regulates insulin levels and triggers enzymes that convert food into energy. Cholesterol from food controls your body's internal cholesterol production and protects your liver. Your liver governs not only how effectively your body burns fat, but it also governs your mood.

Signs of a toxic liver include weight gain, depression, cellulite, abdominal bloating, indigestion, fatigue, mood swings, high blood pressure, elevated cholesterol, and skin rashes. Many people struggle with weight gain and a sluggish metabolism most of their lives, and go through lots of yo-yo dieting unsuccessfully. You might be asking, "Why doesn't anything work?" You may have been tackling the symptom when you should be addressing the cause; weight gain is often due to poor liver function. The liver performs more than four hundred different jobs, and is the body's most important metabolism-enhancing organ. It acts as a filter to clear the body of toxins, metabolize protein, control hormonal balance, and enhance our immune system.

*"Thank you, thank you! With your help, I am off the anti-depressant that I had been taking off and on for almost 20 years. Wow, I can't believe it! I had been convinced that it was something I was going to have to take for the rest of my life. I feel great; I still get a little emotional the week before my period, but it is manageable. In addition to that, I am off the Armour Thyroid. I will have*

*my levels checked again in two months, but the last time it was checked I was holding in the normal range.*

*Also, when I started working with you, I was on the verge of having my gall-bladder out. I am happy to say, I still have my gallbladder with no significant issues. Anyway, thank you again, I know if I had not found you, I would not feel so amazing!*

—Casie

> **HEALTH TIP:** The liver is where T4 is converted to T3, which is the activated thyroid hormone. Excess estrogen blocks production of T3. T4 needs to be converted to activated T3, a process that happens in the liver. T3 is what makes us feel good. A supplement called EstroFactors helps detox this bad estrogen out of the liver, which in turn will heal liver function and increase T3.

Your liver is a "worker bee" that can even regenerate its own damaged cells, but your liver is not invincible. When it is abused and lacks essential nutrients, or when it is overwhelmed by toxins and excess estrogens, it no longer performs as it should. Fat may build up in the liver and just under the skin, hormone imbalances can develop, and toxins can increase and get into the bloodstream. The liver metabolizes not only fats, but also proteins and carbohydrates for fuel. It breaks down amino acids from proteins into various pieces to help build muscle; this process directly impacts your calorie burn. It also transports amino acids through the bloodstream for hormone balance, which is critical to avoid water retention, bloating, cravings, as well other undesired weight issues. There are many different amino acids that have a variety of important jobs. For example, L-tryptophan is an amino acid that comes from protein, which in turn helps build serotonin. Other amino acids also help move waste (like excess "bad" estrogen); detoxification and elimination of this waste occurs through the kidney. These amino acids also perform many other functions, like building muscles.

The liver's most important function, and the one that puts it at greatest risk for damages, is to detoxify the numerous toxins that attack our bodies daily. A healthy liver detoxifies many damaging substances and eliminates them without polluting the bloodstream. When we cleanse the liver and eat the right foods, liver metabolism will improve and we will start burning fat.

> **HEALTH TIP: Speed up liver cleansing with milk thistle and sweating! Sit in a sauna or practice hot yoga. Just make sure to hydrate and refuel your electrolytes afterwards.**

As liver function improves, so does energy. With more energy, fitness improves, because we have the ability to exercise more and improve our muscle tone. If you notice that you are more edgy, easily stressed, have elevated cholesterol, skin irritations, depression, sleep difficulties, indigestion, kidney damage, brain fog, hypothyroidism, chronic fatigue, weight gain, poor memory, PMS, blood sugar imbalances, or allergies, your liver may be to blame. The liver also plays a role in migraines. If this vital organ is overloaded with toxic substances, it can cause inflammation that triggers migraine pain. If you have tried many ways to improve your health and energy level and nothing seemed to help, it is possible that your tired liver is triggering your difficulties. Restoring liver function is one of the most essential actions you could ever do for your health. When the liver gets congested, it will remain that way and get worse until it gets cleaned and revitalized.

The following is a testimonial from a client with many problems including depression:

*When I began my journey, I was size 3X. I had terrible mood swings and depression. I was diagnosed with autoimmune diseases such as fibromyalgia, idiopathic thrombocytic pupurra (ITP), osteoarthritis and asthma. I had fatty liver disease, high blood pressure, eczema, rosacea, skin tags and migraines. I am now an extra large, and I have no depression or mood swings. Though there is no test to prove it, I feel I no longer have fibromyalgia. I no longer use inhalers for asthma and I feel as though that has disappeared, too. The damage from the osteoarthritis unfortunately cannot be reversed. My low blood platelets from the ITP used to average a count of 30,000 and now sit between 70 and 80,000. My iron count averaged around 2 or 3 and I use to get infusions every 6 months. I now average a count of 10 and haven't had an infusion in over 18 months. A recent ultrasound shows my liver is now normal. My blood pressure is stable. Skin tags are gone, eczema flare ups are rare and my rosacea is better. Migraine headaches are a thing of my past. I haven't had a cold in over two years. I have removed 90% of prescription medications from my medicine cabinet. Nobody can convince me that this is a coincidence. I believe 100% there are health benefits to this way of eating.*

*—Terri*

> For 90% of dieters, a deficiency in one of four essential brain chemicals can cause weight gain, fatigue, and stress. The solution to losing weight doesn't lie in deprivation diets; it lies in balancing our neurotransmitters. Specialized nutritionists, like myself, and advanced practitioners are focusing on how the brain affects our health.
>
> 1.  Serotonin influences appetite
>
> 2.  GABA curbs emotional eating
>
> 3.  Acetylcholine regulates fat storage
>
> 4.  Dopamine controls metabolism
>
> When these brain chemicals are balanced, our bodies are more able to lose those extra pounds.

As we all know, being overweight can affect our mood, emotional well-being, and personal and family relationships. But what you don't know is that our brains and neurotransmitter supplies affect food intake, appetite regulation, and energy balance.

Have you ever experienced any of the following: persistent feelings of sadness, irritability, tension, decreased interest or pleasure in usual hobbies, loss of energy, feeling tired despite lack of activity, a change in appetite with significant weight loss or weight gain, a change in sleeping patterns, decreased ability to make decisions or concentrate, feelings of worthlessness, hopelessness, or thoughts of suicide?

I see a lot of these issues with clients and they all can be red flags for depression. It is no wonder that one out of every six Americans will have depression sometime during their lifetime. Although depression is a real medical illness, many people still mistakenly believe it is a personal weakness. That "weakness" is a genuine problem, with roots in your body's brain chemistry. You can take charge of your life again by understanding and taking steps to balance your brain.

Depression has no single cause; often, it results from a combination of factors. Some of the causes may include nutrition, certain diseases or illnesses, family history of depression, difficult life events, certain medications, or excessive alcohol consumption. Whatever the cause, depression is not just a state of mind. It is related to physical changes in the chemicals of the brain. Everything in our bodies including our brain and its chemistry makes us who we are.

Too little or too much of any brain chemical alters our behavior, which can take away our happiness. The combination of these events creates a different personality, and in the end, changes our destiny.

Nourishing our brain fills our heart with reason and compassion; happiness and love; and forgiveness and understanding. It gives us the ability to tolerate all the stress in the world and to appreciate all the beauty in life. With the way food manufacturers have created convenient "food," most of us just do not get enough of each nutrient for days, months, and years at a time. Even though we are filling our bellies with substance, most of us are running a deficiency in many of the nutrients we need in order to make those precious brain chemicals — no wonder there is so much depression.

I had a client who tried everything. High dose of fish oil, probiotics, amino acids, and even had a healthy liver. But it wasn't until he cut out grains that his mood improved. This testimony speaks for itself:

*5 months ago I went grain free and about 2 months ago I was able to start going off all of the medications I was taking for my bipolar disorder. My moods have stabilized and I no longer have severe depression. I wish I had known 23 years ago that if I just cut out grains I could control my disorder, I have been on just about every medication out there and some have left permanent damage to me (lithium carbonate damaged my thyroid and I have to be on medication for the rest of my life). Being grain free & lower carb I've lost 35 lbs. (still need to lose a lot more) I sleep better, and have more energy.*

*Wellbutrin sr 150 mg 2 times a day, Abilify 15 mg 1 time a day, Lamictal 150 mg 2 times a day, Cymbalta 30 mg 3 times a day, Klonopin 1 mg 2 times a day*

*I'm off all those medications now!*

*This is not related to depression but just wanted to add 3 years ago I started having inappropriate sinus tachycardia my heart rate would always be between 130-200 bpm even at rest my Doctors put me on 2 different blood pressure medication to control my heart rate (LOPRESSOR 100MG 3 times a day & DILTIAZEM24HR 240MG 1 time a day) I would faint all the time and 1 time I fractured my foot. It got so bad I had a cardiac loop recorder implanted in my chest and I even went to a Cardiac Electrophysiology (heart rhythm specialist) because they wanted to ablate the sinus node of my heart. In the past few months my heart rate has returned to normal 70-85 bpm without any medication.*

—*Dennis*

Concentration, sleep, energy levels, mood swings, fidgeting, even the ability to sweat are all controlled by essential chemicals in our bodies. Serotonin, dopamine, GABA, and acetylcholine are some of the more important ones; these are strongly influenced by diet, stress, exercise, sunlight, sleep, and other lifestyle factors. Of course, the lifestyle of today is radically different than it was long ago. Consider how these factors from modern life commonly influence us:

HIGH-SUGAR/CARBOHYDRATE AND LOW-FAT DIET. More insulin means a neurotransmitter imbalance and reduced serotonin, GABA, dopamine, and acetylcholine.

BEING INDOORS (LACK OF SUNLIGHT). Reduced melatonin from lack of sunlight disturbs the sleep cycle and cause seasonal depression (also called SAD).

LACK OF SLEEP. Reduced serotonin

STRESS. Reduced serotonin

MODERN FOOD PROCESSING. Consumption of trans-fat, chemical additives, and very little omega-3, Vitamins A, D, E, and K = reduced serotonin, acetylcholine, and dopamine

LACK OF EXERCISE. Decreased serotonin and dopamine

BORING CLASSES OR JOB, LACK OF ACTIVITY. Reduced dopamine and norepinephrine.

Reduced neurotransmitters with high levels of stress, lack of sleep, sunlight, exercise, and poor nutrition are connected with attention deficit disorder (ADD), irritability, depression, aggression, anxiety, lack of concentration, chronic pain, restlessness or fatigue, nausea, obsessive-compulsive disorder, weight gain, fibromyalgia, arthritis, chronic fatigue syndrome, heat intolerance, and other syndromes. For example, fluctuating serotonin levels are connected with bipolar disorder. You don't have to feel depressed or anxious; symptoms may be purely physical and therefore quite treatable.

Reduced dopamine caused by boring surroundings and lack of exercise may manifest as ADD, impulsivity, lack of concentration, restlessness, and depression or loss of pleasure. Dopamine is the "feel good" chemical that illegal drugs mimic; these drugs may include cocaine, heroin, marijuana, as well as non-illegal drugs like cigarettes, coffee, and alcohol. Ritalin and other ADD drugs are found to increase dopamine activity.

Modern food processing has completely altered the types of fatty acids we consume. Since our brain is composed largely of fatty acids, we are missing the "bricks" needed for healthy brain production of acetylcholine. In addition, we are eating lots of man-made chemicals. For example, food coloring is mostly made from petroleum, which isn't nourishing for any parts of our body.

Sugar and carbohydrates elevate insulin levels. High insulin tells the body to store what you just ate as fat, thereby dropping your blood sugar concentration. When you are a "sugar burner," your brain is programmed to only run on sugar, so it thinks it is deprived of food. Poor concentration and depression can result. Also, the low blood sugar makes you hungry, which causes you to eat more sugar or carbohydrates, and the cycle is repeated. Finally, insulin levels affect certain neurotransmitters, such as serotonin. Insulin also changes many other systems throughout the body, including our estrogen and testosterone levels, which determine our output of acetylcholine.

A diet that includes a fat-free Yoplait yogurt for breakfast, a Slim Fast for lunch, and a "Healthy Choice" frozen meal for dinner starves our bodies at the cellular level. Poor nutrition can result in lower levels of brain chemicals, specifically serotonin. Vitamins B6, C, and E (the stress vitamins) are particularly important to consume every day! A well-formulated keto-adapted diet filled with healthy fats will help your brain burn ketones instead of glucose, and you will begin to feel like a new person.

Constant stress requires our bodies to constantly respond. Responding at that rate quickly depletes our bodies and can lead to serious health problems like low mood, anxiousness, sleep difficulties, and weight gain. When your body is constantly "switched on," it never gets the relief it needs. This can lead to changes in the levels of all neurotransmitters. Poor food choices, family issues, work issues, and excess exercise are all stressors on the body.

Neurotransmitters control so many aspects of our well-being. Take this assessment to find out where you may need some extra attention.

# NEUROTRANSMITTER ASSESSMENT

## Serotonin

| Item | True | False |
|---|---|---|
| Eating is a common way that I socialize with others. | | |
| I am a deep-feeling person. | | |
| I am easily irritated. | | |
| I am very suspicious. | | |
| I am extremely artistic. | | |
| I believe my ideas are superior. | | |
| I can easily take advantage of others. | | |
| I can't find meaning in life. | | |
| I can't relax. | | |
| I crave carbohydrates. | | |
| I crave salt. | | |
| I don't do the activities I used to enjoy. | | |
| I drain myself giving to others, but then often fill myself with food. | | |
| I engage in daring activities, such as skydiving. | | |
| I've had thoughts of self-destruction or suicide. | | |
| I find myself thinking about the same things over and over again. | | |
| I have little energy to exercise. | | |
| I have many frivolous relationships. | | |

| Item | True | False |
|---|---|---|
| I just like to "eat, drink, and be merry." | | |
| I need an alcoholic drink in order to get a good night's sleep. | | |
| I need to eat right before going to bed. | | |
| I rarely stick to a plan or agenda. | | |
| I usually grab a quick meal on the run. | | |
| I'm never hungry, although sometimes I find myself eating more than I should. | | |
| I'm not as strong as I use to be. | | |
| I crave carbohydrates and salt. | | |
| I'm not ever very hungry, but still tend to overeat. | | |
| I find it hard to stay asleep through the night. | | |
| I don't do many activities as I use to enjoy. | | |
| I drain myself by giving too much to others. | | |
| I obsess over little things. | | |
| I feel like the world is passing me by. | | |
| I engage in daring activities like skydiving or motorcycle riding. | | |
| I feel emotions more deeply than others. | | |
| Total Number of True Responses | | |

## Dopamine

| Item | True | False |
|---|---|---|
| At parties, I can't control my eating. | | |
| I occasionally experience total exhaustion, without even exerting myself. | | |
| Caffeinated drinks put me in a better mood. | | |
| I am a smoker. | | |
| I am a very domineering person. | | |
| I am eccentric or unconventional. | | |
| I am self-centered. | | |

| Item | True | False |
|---|---|---|
| I am very self-critical. | | |
| I experience bloating after eating. | | |
| I crave sugar frequently. | | |
| I drink more than three alcoholic beverages per week. | | |
| I prefer to eat alone. | | |
| I eat my lunch while I'm working. | | |
| I eat only to re-energize my body. | | |
| I find exercise revitalizing. | | |
| I get easily sad or depressed. | | |
| I am easily irritated. | | |
| I have gained more than 20 pounds since my 20's. | | |
| I have no energy unless I consume caffeine. | | |
| I have trouble getting out of bed in the morning. | | |
| I know I need to exercise, but I tend to put it off. | | |
| I have a low drive to do the things I used to be passionate about. | | |
| I overeat when I am anxious or stressed. | | |
| I tend to be a loner. | | |
| I'm critical of myself, but am even more critical of my friends and family. | | |
| I feel happier after consuming caffeine (coffee, tea, soda, or other uppers). | | |
| I gain weight in the belly. | | |
| I tend to do things differently than others. | | |
| I have little-to-no sex drive. | | |
| I tend to procrastinate. | | |
| I feel fatigued all day, even after a full night's sleep. | | |
| Total Number of True Responses | | |

## GABA

| Item | True | False |
|---|---|---|
| Caffeine has little effect on me. | | |
| I don't have specific food cravings. | | |
| Cooking is one way I like to take care of my loved ones. | | |
| Dinner is not complete without dessert. | | |
| I can create strong, lasting bonds with others. | | |
| I can sense that others want to harm me. | | |
| I often choose the same things to eat. | | |
| I crave bitter foods, if anything. | | |
| I embarrass easily. | | |
| I often drink too much. | | |
| I have experimented with drugs. | | |
| I have fits of anger. | | |
| I like exercise because it helps me relax. | | |
| I lose my temper easily. | | |
| I love to experience new things. | | |
| I need a lot of food to fill me up. | | |
| I often feel tired even when I have had a full night's sleep. | | |
| Sometimes, I overeat. | | |
| I share too much personal information about myself with others. | | |
| I often eat my meals too fast. | | |
| I worry more than I used to. | | |
| I frequently feel nervous and jumpy. | | |
| I'm afraid of conflicts and altercations. | | |
| My thoughts get confused. | | |
| When I make a decision, it's final. | | |
| I frequently experience back pain or muscle tension. | | |
| I am easily perplexed. | | |
| I have had an eating disorder. | | |
| Total Number of True Responses | | |

## Acetylcholine

| Item | True | False |
|---|---|---|
| I am a person who can't get enough of new ideas or experiences. | | |
| I am detail oriented. | | |
| Cheese is a large part of my diet. | | |
| I can't get enough of new drugs or of visiting new places. | | |
| I desire fatty foods. | | |
| I don't like to exercise anymore. | | |
| I eat lots of low-calorie foods like fresh fruits and veggies. | | |
| I experience mood swings. | | |
| I find it more comfortable to do things alone rather than in a large group. | | |
| I am flirtatious. | | |
| I have had an eating disorder at one point in my life. | | |
| I have lost muscle tone. | | |
| I have tried many unconventional, alternative remedies. | | |
| I lack imagination. | | |
| I like to talk about what is troubling me. | | |
| I like to try different cuisines and foods. | | |
| I love stretching my muscles. | | |
| I love yoga. | | |
| I need a lot of nurturing and attention. | | |
| I often feel restless or agitated. | | |
| I tend to see myself in a desirable light. | | |
| Losing weight is a priority to me. | | |
| Dinner is usually accompanied by alcohol or wine. | | |
| Some people describe me as having my "head in the clouds." | | |

| Item | True | False |
|---|---|---|
| By the end of the day, I often forget what I have eaten. | | |
| I love to experience the aromas and the beauty of food. | | |
| I need to write things down to avoid forgetting them. | | |
| I have a dry mouth or dry skin. | | |
| I prefer to be alone rather than in a large group. | | |
| I often feel "on edge." | | |
| I can't get enough of new exciting things.. | | |
| Total Number of True Responses | | |

Once you add up your totals, which area is low (more than fifteen "True" responses)? Serotonin? Dopamine? GABA? Acetylcholine? All of them? No need to worry. Many people have been consuming "substance" instead of "food" for so long that many imbalances often occur. You are in charge now to take the steps to create a healthy brain. Each of the following sections will describe how to balance all your precious neurotransmitters to help you become the fun-loving, balanced person you are.

So what causes neurotransmitter deficiencies? Here are some of the major reasons we can suffer from depressed neurotransmitter levels.

# 1. Dieting and Poor Food Choices: Not Enough Fat!

This is the most common cause of self-induced neurotransmitter deficiencies. Limiting fat intake or choosing popular "fad diets" that endorse their own prepackaged foods in order to lose weight restricts the amounts of basic building blocks (neurotransmitter precursors) needed to produce enough neurotransmitters. Studies from major universities, including Harvard, MIT, and Oxford, have documented that women on low-fat diets significantly deplete their serotonin within three weeks of starting the diet. This induced serotonin deficiency eventually leads to increased cravings, moodiness, and poor motivation. These all contribute to rebound weight gain, the most common, yet unfortunate, consequence of low-fat dieting.

Increasing neurotransmitter production during dieting is strongly encouraged to avoid yo-yo dieting. This is accomplished by taking dietary neurotransmitter precursor supplements during dieting.

## 2. Gluten, Leaky Gut and Neurotransmitters

Patients with depression or anxiety are told they have a chemical imbalance. I have found numerous clients who are suffering from mood disorders to be gluten sensitive. When they eliminate gluten from their life, they become a whole new person. But how could a food cause depression? Let's take a look.

Gluten is the protein found in wheat, rye, barley, and oats. Have you ever put flour and water together to make your own gooey paste? In Poland, they use this for wallpaper paste. I'm not putting that "gummy" paste in my body: it causes way too much inflammation.

Here is a testimony of a client dealing with food allergies and depression:

*The very first time in my life I was asked if I liked myself, I couldn't answer. Yes, I knew I needed to seek help. This was the turning point in my life. I was 17 years old. I first tried traditional medicine: anti-depressants, anxiety medications, thyroid medication for my "hypothyroid" etc. but with little to no avail. I turned to nontraditional medicine. I was 20 years old. I was able to treat my illness through diet and nutrition, but I realize not all cases are that simple. I strongly believe that had I seen a psychologist before my lifestyle change, they would have diagnosed me as bi-polar. I was a mess. Sad, angry, paranoid, blaming others; something was always "wrong" or "a muck" but I never could put a finger on it. I would break down and cry throughout the day and I would always "come up" with a reason why I felt the way I did.*

*I first started by making dietary changes such as eating protein, less grains and less sugar. It helped some, but not enough. I then sought professional help.*

*At my appointment, I started to cry. I said that I don't know what's wrong with me, maybe it's just been a long day. Maybe it's all the testing and pocking and prodding. I remember feeling a dark cloud over me. I was told, "You're having an allergic reaction." I replied, "I am?" This thought gave me hope.*

*Once I started your diet, my cloud was lifted, my brain fog, my depression, my pain, my suffering. I was a "new person." I was my old self again! I was 21 years old.*

*After the lifestyle changes of diet and nutrition, my fibromyalgia, freezing cold all the time, and sadness went away. Things were finally "perfected" once I went 100% gluten free. Until I went 100% gluten free I kept developing new allergies. I was always bloated and constipated. I would still have occasional emotional unsteadiness.*

*With Maria's guidance of supplements and staying 100% compliant to her diet, my gut has finally healed, my emotional health completely stabilized, my acne gone, excess pounds gone, brain fog gone, and my tired / fatigue is gone. I am the healthy image I longed to be. It took time, persistence, patience, and self-discipline. It has been a journey that has paid off! I am now a wife and mother of three and have the positive energy they all need. I can truly be the sound and encouraging spiritual head of the home, focused on them and not on myself. I am now 29 years old.*

—*Lacy*

After the digestive tract, the most commonly affected system to be irritated by gluten is the nervous system. It is thought that gluten causes depression in one of two ways. Gluten causes inflammation in the body. A gluten-sensitive individual's immune system responds to the protein gliadin. Unfortunately, that protein is similar in structure to other proteins present in the body, including those in the brain and nerve cells. A cross reactivity can occur where the immune system "confuses" all proteins in the body for the protein gliadin. This is called cellular mimicry, where the body attacks its own tissues, and inflammation results.

When inflammation happens in the brain and nervous system, a variety of symptoms can occur, including depression. Research shows us that patients with symptoms involving the nervous system suffer from digestive problems only 13% of the time. This is significant because mainstream medicine equates gluten sensitivity almost exclusively with digestive complaints. Please note that even though most doctors will dismiss a gluten allergy or sensitivity if you don't have any digestive issues, this is not true. You can have problems with gluten that show up in other parts of your body, not just the digestive track. Gluten can attack any organ: thyroid, gallbladder, nervous system, joints (arthritis), cellular membrane (multiple sclerosis), you name it.

In a study examining blood flow to the brain, patients with untreated celiac disease were compared to patients treated with a gluten-free diet for a year. The findings were amazing. In the untreated group, 73% of the patients had abnormalities in blood circulation of the brain, while only 7% of patients in the treated group showed any abnormalities. The patients with the circulation problems were frequently suffering from anxiety and depression as well.

In addition to finding circulation problems, other research looks at the association between gluten sensitivity and its interference with protein absorption. Specifically, the amino acid tryptophan (which we learned about in chapter 1), is essential for brain health. Tryptophan is a protein in the brain responsible for the feelings of well-being and relaxation. A deficiency in this protein can be correlated to feelings of depression and anxiety. Ninety percent of serotonin production occurs in the digestive tract. So, it makes sense that food might have an effect, either positive or negative, on serotonin production.

Our society is too willing to accept a "chemical imbalance" as an explanation for their symptoms. Instead of getting to the root cause of the condition, we simply swallow a pill — a pill that, in the case of anti-depressants, has very dangerous and undesired side effects.

The frequency with which clients can taper off their anti-depressants is considered "unbelievable" to many mainstream doctors, yet it happens regularly. How is that possible? Well, it is important to look at the root cause of the depression, rather than just putting a "Band-Aid" over the problem. Instead, I find success with a gluten-free diet as the main path to recovery, along with a therapeutic dose of amino acids, such as 5-HTP or GABA as well as vitamin B and other key nutrients.

Food allergies can also affect our children's behavior. Encounters with allergens stimulate the release of serotonin and histamine from most cells in the body. This stimulation alters arousal, attention, activity, and vigilance. As a result, a highly allergic child can be either quite sluggish or quite hyperactive, depending upon the system of the allergic reaction. Eliminating all allergens from the diet will eliminate hyperactivity or lethargy and inattention.

The increase in celiac disease might be because there is more gluten being consumed: "gluten enteropathy" is another term for this illness. Gluten is useful in cooking because it promotes a resistant, chewy feel to a lot of foods, including baked goods. But, as we increase our consumption of "convenient" foods (such as pizza, granola bars, and cereal) we increase the amount of gluten-containing grains on a daily basis.

When I tell clients to eat "gluten free" they often grab all the "gluten free" prepackaged foods on the shelf, but that most likely will cause more mood issues and weight gain and will slow the healing process in your gut. Rice flour, the common flour substitute in gluten-free products, is higher in calories, higher in carbohydrates, and lower in nutrients than regular flour. It can cause more inflammation in our body. So my recommendation is to make your own healthier options by using almond flour and coconut flour, which are very easy to digest. The healthy fats in nuts are actually nourishing to our brain. Nuts are also filled with iron. After first being diagnosed with a gluten allergy, you may feel tired; this is linked to an iron deficiency.

Gluten is the first allergy I look at when there are signs of a food allergy, but there are other common food allergies to look at as well. Dairy, soy, eggs, and fructose are all food allergies that can cause the same issues as gluten. If you suspect an allergy, you have two options: you can either eliminate certain foods for a two-month period to see what happens to your body and brain, or you can get a stool analysis to test for specific allergies. I find that most people stick to an allergen-free diet if they have the results sitting in front of them, verifying that there is definitely an allergy. Stool tests are not cheap, but are a lot more accurate than blood tests. Blood tests are 70 percent inaccurate. My suggestion is to invest in your well-being and get tested.

If you discover that you are allergic or sensitive to gluten and you don't know where to begin, all the recipes in my books are gluten-free.

## 3. Hormone Imbalances

Hormones influence neurotransmitter release and activity. If hormones are deficient or are off balance, neurotransmitters do not function well. Premenstrual Syndrome (PMS) is a classic example of how low serotonin levels can temporarily shift each month. Mood, appetite, and sleep can be severely disrupted one to two weeks before the menstrual cycle. Another neurotransmitter, acetylcholine, decreases during menopause when dramatic changes in memory, mood, energy, sleep, weight, and sexual desire occur.

HEALTH TIP: Women experience more depression than men because men have more tryptophan than women do. There are three types of estrogen our body can make:
1. Ovaries produce healthy estrogen (estradiol)
2. Fat cells store and form unhealthy estrogen (estrone)
3. The third type is produced only when pregnant (estriol)

Healthy estrogen from our ovaries gives women ample curves, attractive breasts, and youthful skin. However, estrogen from our fat cells and external sources causes too many curves (you might call them "bulges") mainly in the belly area (men can have bad estrogen, too). Farmers have known this for years. They use a little synthetic estrogen to fatten their cattle.

Estrogen activates an enzyme called hepatic tryptophan 2,3 dioxygenase that shifts the metabolism of tryptophan from building serotonin (happy) to creating kynurenic (depression). Women already have lower serum levels of tryptophan than men do, which is part of the reason why we are more vulnerable to depression and the overconsumption of carbohydrates in the first place. If you are also consuming gluten and fructose, it lowers the already less available tryptophan, which further increases depression.

Saturated fat produces healthy hormones. Low-fat, low-cholesterol diets can be very unhealthy, especially for women. All our major hormones are made from cholesterol: estrogen, progesterone, cortisol, DHEA, and testosterone. If we don't eat enough, our bodies divert cholesterol from our endocrine system to use for brain function and repair. When that happens, it's almost impossible for our bodies to maintain hormonal balance. Hot flashes, here we come!

# 4. Prolonged Emotional or Physical Stress

The human body is programmed to handle sudden, acute, and short bouts of stress. On the other hand, prolonged, chronic stress takes a toll on the "fight or flight" stress hormones and neurotransmitters. Eventually, these become depleted and coping becomes more difficult. If you have ever heard of "adrenal fatigue," this is a terrible snowball effect for weight gain and emotional issues.

> **HEALTH TIP:** Have you ever looked at the roasted almonds you grab for a "healthy" snack from the vending machine? I bet you would find MSG in the ingredients. MSG, an excitotoxin, causes damage to the neurons in your brain and has links to Parkinson's disease, Alzheimer's, Huntington's disease, and many others. Children are very susceptible to this type of effect on their sensitive and growing brains. Excitotoxins essentially overexcite the neurons in the brain; the neurons become exhausted and die.
>
> Neurotoxins are also a main cause of seizures, though the damage may not be seen until many years later. When this happens, our neurotransmitters responsible for focus, mood, and memory have a hard time finding and recognizing their receptors due to the inflammation of the membranes in the brain cells caused by the consumption of MSG. Consuming MSG triples the amount of insulin the pancreas creates.
>
> Brain levels of the neurotransmitter dopamine (important for mood and focus) are lowered by 95% when you ingest excitotoxins. But what is even more disturbing is that when you switch to being 100% free of processed food, your brain remains unable to produce normal amounts of dopamine in the hippocampus (the part of the brain most responsible for consolidating memory). This is one reason for the high rates of ADHD and depression.

# 6. Abnormal Sleep

Many neurotransmitters responsible for proper sleep, especially serotonin, are produced during REM sleep (around 3 to 4 hours after you have fallen asleep). Serotonin converts to melatonin, the sleep hormone. When serotonin levels are low, melatonin levels will also be low. When this happens, disrupted sleep occurs and less neurotransmitters are produced, causing a vicious cycle.

# 7. Medications

Long-term use of acne medications, diet pills, stimulants, pain pills, narcotics, and recreational drugs can deplete neurotransmitter stores and damage our liver. The use of ma huang (also called ephedra) and prescription diet pills use up large amounts of dopamine and serotonin. This can result in "rebound" appetite control problems, sluggish metabolism, low energy, and an unsteady mood.

# 8. Neurotoxins

Heavy metal toxicity, cleaning agents, hair chemicals, pesticides, fertilizers, industrial solvents, and recreational drugs cause damage to neurons and decrease neurotransmitter production. Excess caffeine, nicotine, and alcohol can also be neurotoxic. The street drug, Ecstasy, has highly detrimental neurotoxic effects. It can completely drain serotonin and permanently damage neurons, making recovery impossible.

# 9. Genetic Predisposition

Some people are born with a limited ability to make adequate amounts of neurotransmitters. They display symptoms of a deficiency as children and often have relatives who suffered from noteworthy appetites and mental illnesses. As they get older, affected individuals experience even more intense symptoms and debilitation.

# 10. Candida or Yeast Overgrowth

An overgrowth of yeast causes extreme sugar cravings and low good gut bacteria. Our moods come from our gut. Killing the yeast is essential to healing our brain chemistry and increasing moods.

Below is a list of the roles of neurotransmitters and their importance in the nervous system and how they affect the entire human body:

- Emotionally
  - Mood and feelings
  - Social attitude
  - Actions or behavior
- Mentally
  - Motivation
  - Learning ability
  - Focus and mental clarity
- Physically
  - Weight gain
  - Energy levels
  - Cardiac health
  - Sleep

## SEROTONIN: CONTROL CRAVINGS

*Hi Maria,*

*I just want to tell everyone what a difference you've made in not only my family's life, but in my patients' lives, too. As a doctor, I was always pushing "healthy whole grains" and fruits like bananas for potassium, but after looking at myself in the mirror, I knew something wasn't right with this idea of calories in and calories out. I was eating a very clean diet of "healthy whole grains," quinoa and tons of fruit, but I was overweight, had adult acne and was feeling a bit depressed. And I had anxiety when it came to food; counting "points" was not working for me.*

*One of my patients gave me a copy of your book, and I was so inspired that I decided to do a phone consult, which forever changed my life. I have to be honest, the first week was awful. I felt like one of my patients suffering from drug withdrawal, but I now understand that the sugars and grains were my drug. Your explanation of how the protein in the wheat (similar to other proteins in the body), which was causing cellular mimicry in my nervous system and brain, was also causing my slight depression; it made total sense. You taught me that I was gluten sensitive; this, too, was shocking to me since I didn't suffer from any intestinal issues. But after working with you for six weeks, I no longer felt depressed! Not only that, but I lost 31 pounds and no longer had to use my topical medication for adult acne (but after watching your cosmetics tutorial video, I realized how toxic those products were to my liver, which also contributed to my poor moods and inability to lose weight).*

*You not only changed my life, but my kids are now 100% grain free and enjoy picking out recipes from your kids cookbook for snacks at school. I also feel so much better about setting a good example for my patients. I had felt uncomfortable preaching to them about what to eat while being overweight. Now I know the whole truth and I am forever grateful. The consult with you really changed my life more than you will ever realize.*

*—Dr. Sally*

Clients with adequate serotonin are happy and live in the moment. Despite being calm, they can be spontaneous and seek a wide variety of exciting new activities. Serotonin is produced within the occipital lobe, the area of the brain that regulates sight. Serotonin is connected with mood, drive, ambition, decision making, and the ability to experience pleasure. Research in the *American Journal of Science* suggests that low levels of this brain chemical can cause psychological symptoms like depression, impulsivity, suspiciousness, shortsightedness, or aggressiveness. Fortunately, increasing levels of serotonin quickly improves confidence, restores rationality, and boosts feelings of happiness.

Serotonin is used mainly in your gut; about 80 to 90% is found there, and the rest is found in our brain. This is why what we eat is so important. Serotonin does various things like control appetite, hormones, sleep, mood, and anger. Serotonin deficiency is a primary cause of depression. It is one of the more well-studied neurotransmitters because it affects our personality in such a profound way. Serotonin is the brain's natural antidepressant and regulator of sleep, mood, and appetite.

The other neurotransmitters discussed in this chapter allow communication between two neurons. Serotonin, on the other hand, alters the efficiency of communication between neurons that may use a variety of other chemicals as their primary neurotransmitter.

As it is with all neurotransmitters, there needs to be a balance in serotonin levels in order for this powerful substance to be processed properly. Excessive amounts of serotonin may cause relaxation, sedation, and a decrease in sexual drive. Inadequate amounts of serotonin in the brain can amount to debilitating psychiatric conditions such as anxiety disorders, depression, and obsessive-compulsive mood disorders.

Other symptoms of low serotonin can include constipation, carbohydrate cravings, premenstrual syndrome, eating disorders, allergies, arthritis, backache, constipation, diarrhea, headache, migraines, insomnia, premature ejaculation, tinnitus, yawning, lack of pleasure, being a loner, perfectionism, rage, shyness, lack of concentration, and slow reactions. It is also important to note that women are often low in serotonin during menstrual cycles, causing cravings, migraines, sleep issues and constipation.

Some people may be born with inherently low serotonin levels, which causes the neuroreceptors to become more sensitive. This in turn may result in higher highs and lower lows, and an increased vulnerability to depression and high carbohydrate cravings early in life.

Prescription medications such as Prozac indirectly raise serotonin levels at the receptor sites by preventing the body from reabsorbing the serotonin, allowing serotonin to go directly to the receptor site that is low in serotonin. This improves mood and well-being, but not without severe side effects. Following the food suggestions and alternative supplements I have provided in this book can greatly enhance serotonin levels without any adverse effects.

Low serotonin levels cause the body to crave carbohydrates and sweets. Carbohydrates will increase insulin in our bloodstream. Insulin will then reward us with an extreme feeling of gratification, which our brain is screaming for, but not for long. Soon after the carbohydrate binge, our serotonin level will diminish and the cycle will continue. Eating these foods in an attempt to relieve the cravings leads to weight gain, which can also cause depression. Following a keto-adapted allergen-free diet will increase serotonin without sacrificing our waistline.

The role of serotonin in weight fluctuation is not straightforward. The connections between serotonin, appetite, and eating disorders are very complicated. For example, in some situations with eating disorders, the receptors for serotonin may be altered. So the "fix" is not necessarily to simply raise serotonin levels. There may be other aspects of the serotonin chemical pathway—the receptors, transporters, and metabolism—that are not functioning in a normal way, including our hormone ghrelin.

When levels of this brain chemical are low, the body never gets the signal that it needs to shut down and recharge for the next day. This leaves the brain tired and triggers the release of ghrelin, a hormone that stimulates appetite, in order to increase energy levels. That's why women with low levels of serotonin often experience intense carbohydrate and salt cravings that make it difficult to avoid the overeating that can cause weight gain.

Researchers at the UT Southwestern Medical Center found that serotonin activates the nerves that curb appetite while simultaneously deactivating the nerves that increase appetite. In fact, Fen-Phen, a weight loss drug banned from US markets in 2007 due to cardiac side effects, worked by increasing serotonin release between nerve cells of the brain.

Serotonin is what neuroscientists call a modulator. Serotonin is like a volume control in the brain and nervous system. Antidepressants work by enhancing its availability, while other medications can lower its level and cause depression. Instead of running to your doctor for a prescription drug that is filled with side effects, why not try to change your nutrition first? Nutrition plays a huge role in the function of serotonin.

## Migraines and Serotonin

Does your head ever pound like someone is trying to flatten it with a cement truck? Has it ever hurt so bad your vision has blurred? And why is everyone talking so loud? All you can do is find the quiet place to lie down. You know that no matter who needs you, what deadlines you have, or where you are supposed to be, you won't be there until tomorrow ... you're having another migraine.

A migraine is your body's way of telling you that something is wrong. Approximately one out of every ten Americans experience migraines, with women being affected three times more often than men. This painful headache is most commonly experienced between the ages of 15 and 55, and 70 to80% of sufferers have a family history of migraine. Symptoms may be (but are not limited to) intense throbbing (often on one side of the head only), visual disturbances, nausea, vomiting, diarrhea, increased sensitivity to light, sounds and smells, stiffness of the neck and shoulders, tingling or stiffness in the limbs, and an inability to concentrate.

A variety of factors can trigger a migraine. Triggers include alteration of sleep–wake cycle; food allergies or food sensitivities; food additives; a blood sugar imbalance; medications that cause a swelling of the blood vessels; daily or near daily use of medications designed for relieving headache attacks; bright lights; sunlight; fluorescent lights; TV and movie viewing; and excessive noise.

But that's not all — low serotonin can cause a migraine. This is why during a woman's menstrual cycle, estrogen and progesterone levels shift too fast, causing a massive drop in serotonin and triggering a migraine. Research has linked migraine headaches with imbalances in our neurotransmitters, specifically serotonin.

The following is a testimonial from a client who had mood issues:

*I have been on meds for anxiety and depression for almost seven years. Even though I never really thought they made a difference, I just kept taking them. For eight years! I decided on my 37th birthday that I was done. I stopped all of my prescript meds cold turkey, against my doctor's advice. I am now about six weeks in, and I have never felt better and more in control. I sleep great and I can't stop telling people about it. GABA, 5-HTP, magnesium and going sugar/grain free seem to have done the trick for me, along with a few other things Maria recommended. This is the new me ... and I think it will only get better from here!*

—*Nicole*

## Production of Serotonin

Tryptophan is a naturally occurring substance that can be found in a variety of foods. This substance is a precursor to serotonin and can act as a mild sedative on the human body. It has been shown that transmitters' levels are sensitive to dietary intake. If levels of tryptophan are raised through various forms of food in the diet, it is possible to increase serotonin levels.

Tryptophan must enter the brain by crossing the blood-brain barrier. This barrier, made of brain capillary walls, prevents the passage of bacteria, viruses, and some drugs, yet permits glucose and amino acids to pass through.

Tryptophan attaches itself to receptors on the blood-brain barrier that transport large neutral amino acids (also called LNAA). High blood concentration of LNAA competes with tryptophan, reducing its availability in the brain. A high tryptophan-to-LNAA ratio is more significant than total tryptophan. Meals that increase the ratio increase serotonin production and improve sleep and mood.

Foods with a high tryptophan-to-LNAA ratio are eggs, Parmesan cheese, cheddar cheese, pork chops, caribou, turkey, and quality whey protein. The commercially available alpha-lactalbumin, a whey protein and the primary protein in human breast milk, has a high tryptophan-to-LNAA ratio. Protein powders made from whey protein concentrate or isolate have a high tryptophan-to-LNAA ratio as well. Tryptophan is available as a prescription drug and as a non-prescription supplement. The supplement dose used in clinical studies is 2 to 4 grams daily. It is important to note that if there is a dairy allergy, whey protein and cheese—even though high in tryptophan—should be avoided.

Exercise and sleep patterns also change the levels of serotonin in the brain. Electrical activity of serotonin in the brain increases during physical activity. Serotonin and dopamine levels increase in the blood during exercise.

Serotonin levels fluctuate rhythmically, on a circadian 24-hour cycle. This fluctuation is regulated by the day–night cycle, such that interruptions in the normal period of sleep or activity could disrupt the normal serotonin rhythm. In order to ensure the most consistent cycling of serotonin, hormones, and other neurotransmitters that are regulated in a circadian fashion, consistent sleep patterns are crucial.

To produce more serotonin, aim to get at least two daily servings of animal protein like poultry, eggs, and shrimp per day. Each serving of these foods provides the body with about 300 mg of tryptophan, the amino acid needed to produce serotonin. If you are not on an anti-depressant, adding in a 5-HTP supplement increases serotonin before bed (see list of supplements). It converts tryptophan into serotonin during the sleep cycle. Researchers at the University of Cambridge in the United Kingdom found that a daily dose of 500 mg boosted levels of serotonin within two weeks. **Note:** Some people have a hard time converting 5-HTP to tryptophan, in that case, I recommend taking L-tryptophan.

Below is a list of the best food sources for tryptophan. The list is in descending order of how much you get from a typical portion.

- Sleep (not food, but important)
- Wild game
- Pork
- Avocado
- Egg
- Duck
- Whey protein (if you're not dairy sensitive)
- Turkey
- Sausage
- Halibut
- Beef liver
- Chicken
- Cinnamon
- Chocolate (unsweetened cocoa)

## Supplements for Serotonin

VITAMIN-D (5000 IU) This will provide energy, so take it in the morning. It also elevates mood and contributes to your body's ability to lose fat. **Note:**

Get your vitamin D levels checked. If they are too high, it can cause an inability to sleep.

MELATONIN (1–10 mg) Take this in the evening. It suppresses body weight and visceral fat accumulation the next day. I recommend melatonin patches for best absorption.

5-HTP (200–500 mg) Take this in the evening. It reduces appetite, increases REM sleep, and promotes weight loss. Take with food during the day to avoid daytime sleepiness. I strongly prefer this to L-tryptophan because it crosses the blood-brain barrier much better and you need far less of it. If you suffer from depression, you can take this on an empty stomach in the morning in addition to taking it the evening. This will help your depression but may make you sleepy. **Note:** Do not take 5-HTP with a prescription antidepressant. Getting off antidepressants is tough; I have many clients transitioning right now. I would recommend a personal consultation on how to transition.

OMEGA-3(EPA/DHA) (1000–3000 mg) Take 3 times a day at each meal. High levels increase fat loss and reduce appetite.

MAGNESIUM GLYCINATE (400–1000 mg) Take this in the evening to increase sleep. It also reduces chocolate cravings. Magnesium is a precursor to making serotonin.

ACETYL-L-CARNITINE (500–5000 mg) Take this in the morning. It is an antioxidant that prevents inflammation and increases memory.

DHEA (10–25 mg) This is a "fountain-of-youth" hormone that decreases in the body with age. **Note:** Get your levels checked before taking it.

PHENYLALANINE (500–1000 mg) Taken in the morning, it can balance low-serotonin with more dopamine: this nutrient can be converted to tyrosine, which is converted to dopamine, providing energy.

SAM-E (400–1600 mg) Taken in the morning, it is the first metabolite of the essential amino acid, l-methionine.

TRYPTOPHAN (500–1000 mg) Taken in the evening, it can increase the effectiveness of antidepressants and provide additional serotonin. **Note:** Do not take tryptophan with a prescription antidepressant. Getting off antidepressants is tough, but I have many clients that successfully transition off medications. I would recommend a personal consultation on how to transition.

PROBIOTICS (1 billion per day) Acidophilus and bifidobacteria balance brain chemistry. Take 5 to 15 minutes before meals.

## GABA: CONTROL EMOTIONAL EATING

Anxiety affects approximately 19 million adults in the US. It is highly treatable, yet only one third of those suffering from anxiousness receive treatment.

Maybe you see your anxiousness as something you must endure, something about yourself that is unchangeable. Is it because you think being a "worry wart" or "crabby" are just personality traits like "bubbly" and "happy go lucky"?

If you are having emotional symptoms, you may be experiencing one of the many types of anxiousness. These symptoms include excessive worry; recurring thoughts that reflect exaggerated fears; fears of dying; fears of losing control; irrational worries about being judged or embarrassed; the "reliving" of a traumatic event; and the avoidance of everyday, common situations.

Have you ever had feelings of jumpiness? This is because anxiousness can also be accompanied by physical symptoms, such as muscular aches, sleep difficulties, irritability, trembling, dizziness, heart palpitations, chest pains, sweating, routine compulsions, and poor concentration. The most common physical symptom I see in clients with anxiety is emotional or stress eating.

Each of these different types of anxiousness can be linked to imbalances in a brain neurotransmitter called GABA (gamma-aminobutyric acid). Being a "worry wart" is not a personality trait, it is a physical problem with real answers.

Fifty percent of people have GABA-dominant natures (an imbalance of too much GABA in their system). GABA-natured people are sociable and remain calm amongst chaos. They love organization and are dependable. People with GABA-dominant natures don't have wild mood swings and love team or group activities.

GABA is the brain's natural calming agent. It regulates the nervous system, ensuring brain signals travel from the brain throughout the body in a steady flow. Low levels of GABA can cause feelings of nervousness and shakiness because electrical signals are being sent in short pulses rather than in steady streams. While a balanced brain receives regular, smooth electrical impulses, a GABA-deficient one receives them in spurts. As a result, the brain experiences arrhythmia, or dysrhythmia, which directly affects overall emotional well-being.

People with low levels of GABA are in a constant state of anxiety that increases the desire for food and can trigger binging. Plus, this condition can cause stress-related physical symptoms and muscle aches. Studies also show that GABA shortfalls elevate levels of the stress hormone cortisol, which can contribute to the storage of fat in the belly and will eventually burn out our adrenal levels. This decreases our ability to deal with everyday stressors, and the cycle continues.

GABA is the primary neurotransmitter in the temporal lobe, the area of the brain that governs perception, attention, speech, and motions. Low levels of this chemical have been linked to psychological symptoms such as insecurity, excessive worrying, fear of new experiences, poor concentration, ADD, ADHD, and a lack of impulse control. But as GABA shortfalls are corrected, we can regain calmness, dependability, and objectivity. A GABA deficiency appears in the following symptoms: anxiousness, nervousness, irritability, restlessness, allergies, blurred vision, clammy hands, butterflies in the stomach, dizziness, irritable bowel syndrome, constipation, neuropathy, fibromyalgia, headache, insomnia, trembling or shaking, tinnitus, manic depression, and mood disorders. However, you don't need to have all of these issues in order to be deficient in GABA.

As one of the primary neurotransmitters in the brain, GABA is an inhibitory (rather than an excitatory) chemical responsible for creating the calming, rhythmic electrical impulses in the brain. It elevates the production of alpha waves associated with feeling relaxed (without feeling drowsy) and boosts mental alertness. GABA lowers beta waves, which are impulses that contribute to a state of nervousness, racing thoughts, binge eating, and hyperactivity.

## Ways to Naturally Increase GABA

To avoid taking prescription anti-anxiety medications and dosing in prescriptions such as Xanax, Ativan, or Valium, consider the following natural alternatives:

EAT A KETO-ADAPTED DIET. A ketogenic diet induces epigenetic changes, which stimulate the energetic output of our mitochondria, reduce the production of damaging free radicals, and favor the production of GABA. Ketosis reduces the toxic effects of excitatory pathways in our brains.[55]

EAT FERMENTED VEGETABLES. GABA in food often is synthesized by using lactobacillus and monascus, so several fermented foods contain it. Korean kimchi contains high amounts of good gut bacteria.

ADD IN A B-COMPLEX AT BREAKFAST. Vitamin B boosts GABA production. The amino acid L-glutamine, which the body uses to synthesize GABA, also boosts GABA production.

**GABA SUPPLEMENTS PROMOTE RELAXATION AND SLEEP.** They may also have a role to play in preventing seizures and relieve chronic pain.

**LOAD UP ON GREEN TEA.** Swap coffee for a cup of green or oolong tea. When we feel overworked and worn out, coffee is a natural go-to. But its high levels of caffeine send the activating brain chemical dopamine soaring. The trade-off for short-term productivity is a jittery feeling and insomnia hours later. Try oolong tea instead. It contains GABA, and sipping it may provide you with the break your brain and body needs. The break you'll get may provide you with the stamina to get everything done without feeling worn out.

Green tea contains the anxiety-reducing amino acid L-theanine, which is involved in the formation of GABA. You will, however, have to drink large amounts to obtain any affect. Most green tea sold in the United States contains less than 10 mg of L-theanine, while the suggested dose to decrease symptoms is 50–200 mg.

**SUPPLEMENT WITH THE AMINO ACID L-THEANINE IN ADDITION TO GABA SUPPLEMENTS.** L-theanine is more effective than GABA supplements in crossing the blood-brain barrier.

**ELIMINATE UNNECESSARY STRESS.** Do not train for a marathon if you are dealing with multiple stressors in your life.

**MEDITATE OR TAKE A YOGA CLASS.** These are tasks that can be very difficult at first for those who are low in GABA.

If you're one of the millions who suffer from anxiety or depression, consider amino acids as a safe alternative to reaching for Valium or Prozac. These protein building blocks may be the key to reversing long-standing anxiety and depression. Even better, you don't get the serious side effects commonly associated with pharmaceutical medications. These side effects can typically include a decrease in metabolism, blurred vision, increased heart rate, low blood pressure, nausea, headaches, constipation, memory loss, impaired concentration, and brain fog. In contrast, the clinical use of amino acids produces no side effects or health risks and generates better, longer-lasting healing results.

GABA supplements have also been proposed for improving concentration in attention deficit hyperactivity disorder (ADHD) and promoting prostate health. Specifically, GABA supplements may help to promote sound sleep. GABA participates in promoting relaxation, which explains why many well-known anxiety medications, such as Valium, target GABA receptors in the brain. But unlike many prescription tranquilizers, GABA is not addictive.

**HEALTH TIP:** Flushing out toxins and mercury in your body is essential to mental well-being. Do you have mercury dental fillings?

GABA itself does not cause drowsiness. Instead, by easing anxiety, it simply makes it easier to fall asleep. Some research indicates that the popular insomnia-fighting herb, valerian root (found in "Sleepy Time" tea), boosts GABA levels, too. When treating sleep disorders, some people have the best results when rotating GABA with valerian or melatonin.

GABA supplements can also alleviate stress by calming and stabilizing the brain. Persistent stress also contributes to depression, and evidence shows that GABA has mood-elevating properties. It levels out emotions and provides a stable mood.

GABA also combats chronic pain. Stress can aggravate pain, making you feel worse. As a natural stress-reducer, GABA supplements can help to alleviate the intensity of pain and also diminish pain-related nerve impulses.

The more GABA-producing foods you eat, the more GABA you will be able to create. According to an article posted on *Supplement News*, the highest concentrations of naturally occurring GABA are found in fish, particularly mackerel.

The term "comfort food" takes on new meaning when referring to foods that stimulate the production of this calming chemical in the brain. People with low GABA levels can reduce their anxiety, increase mental focus, and lower irritability without the use of prescriptions by drinking green tea, supplementing with L-theanine, and adding foods high in glutamine to their daily diet. But some people may be so low for so long due to a diet filled with packaged foods that are devoid of glutamine that supplementing GABA or L-glutamine is necessary for getting our brains to function properly.

## GLUTAMINE FOODS:

Cabbage, shrimp, green tea, oolong tea, beef liver, fish, meats, poultry, walnuts, broccoli, spinach, cherry tomatoes, almonds, tree nuts, and fermented vegetables such as kimchi, fermented pickles, and fermented sauerkraut.

## VITAMIN B FOODS:

Halibut, liver, beef, tuna, avocado, turkey, chili peppers, garlic, chili powder, tumeric, paprika, tarragon, dill, basil, marjoram, sage, spearmint, rosemary, oregano, bay leaves, alfalfa, cauliflower, broccoli, kale, spinach, and nuts.

## Supplements to Increase GABA:

INOSITOL (100–10,000 mcg) Produces a calming and relaxing effect by activating GABA.

BRANCHED-CHAIN AMINO ACIDS (5–20 g) Work as a fuel source for muscles and help with physical exertion.

GABA (75–1,000 mg) Controls anxiety that leads to overeating.

TAURINE (500–10,000 mg) May inhibit weight gain.

MAGNESIUM GLYCINATE (400–1000 mg) Increases energy production and is a natural muscle relaxant.

**L-THEANINE** (100–500 mg) Reduces mental and physical stress and produces feelings of relaxation (found in tea).

**L-GLUTAMINE** (4–15 grams per day) This is a fantastic amino acid and is the most abundant in the muscle and blood plasma. It makes up an astounding 61% of your muscle tissue. It's one of the most studied amino acids and it has numerous benefits, but for our purposes here it will increase your GABA levels. It is also a potent growth hormone releaser.

**B-COMPLEX** (500–1000 mg per day) B vitamins are our natural stress relieving vitamins. Most prescription drugs deplete these essential vitamins from our body. It is best to take two doses separately throughout the day since you can only absorb so much of the vitamin at a time.

## ACETYLCHOLINE: DECREASE FAT STORAGE

Acetylcholine controls the brain's speed and mental processes, keeping memory sharp and physical movements quick and precise. Acetylcholine controls activity in the parietal lobe, the area of the brain responsible for processing sensory information, learning, memory and awareness. Inadequate levels of this chemical can cause characteristics like forgetfulness, difficulty prioritizing tasks and an inability to relate to others. Acetylcholine natures enjoy activities involving words, ideas, and communication. Counselors, instructors, artists, writers, and actors are likely to have high acetylcholine levels.

For most women who are predisposed to an acetylcholine deficiency, these symptoms set in with perimenopause. Estrogen and testosterone stimulate the production of acetylcholine. As levels of those hormones decline, so does the production of this brain chemical. This decline prompts symptoms like memory lapses, dry skin, and weight gain.

Acetylcholine deficiency can spur Alzheimer's, multiple sclerosis, dementia, dry mouth, dry skin, reading or writing disorders, speech problems, slow movement, mood swings, learning disorders, verbal memory problems, memory lapses, attention problems, difficulty concentrating, carelessness, and decreased creativity. When acetylcholine deficits are corrected, most people experience increased mental clarity, greater creativity, quicker thinking, and improved empathy.

In the late 1930s, scientists discovered that tissue from the pancreas contained a substance called choline, which helps prevent fatty build-up in the liver and produces acetylcholine. Since then, research has shown that choline is not only found in the pancreas and liver, but is also a huge component of every human cell.

> **Health Tip: Choline helps to transport fat and cholesterol to your cells, thereby preventing the accumulation of fat and cholesterol in your liver. A sign of a choline deficiency is a fatty liver.**

Choline is named after the Greek word meaning bile, which is very appropriate. Bile is produced in the liver; its primary job is making fat compatible with water so that fat-based matter can get transported through the body in our water-based blood. Interestingly, choline has very comparable fat-modifying effects on our cellular membrane. The reason that choline decreases fat storage is because it allows our cell membranes to operate with greater flexibility in handling both fat- and water-soluble molecules. In other words, without choline, fat-based nutrients and waste products could not pass in and out of our cells. Therefore, healthy fats can't get into our cells to make our brain healthy, our skin soft, and our cells happy, and we can't get the stored toxic fat out.

Choline is a key component of the fat-containing structures in cell membranes. Since cell membranes are almost entirely made up of fats, the membranes' health depends on adequate amounts of choline. In the brain, these fat-like molecules are responsible for a very high percentage of total solids, so choline is predominantly important for brain health and its use in brain disorders is immense.

To produce more acetylcholine, eat three servings of choline-rich foods, like eggs (I'm talking about the yolks here … "Egg Beaters" don't count). Free-range, organic eggs are the most beneficial. Free-range chickens with a diet of bugs produce eggs that contain a very high level of healthy omega-3s compared to store-bought eggs. Omega-3 will also stimulate a happier brain by assisting cells in their communication ("happy cells are talking cells"). For example, one of the problems with multiple sclerosis is that cells aren't able to communicate with each other.

Coconut oil, avocados, fish, and nuts will also increase acetylcholine. These foods provide high doses of vitamin B (related to choline), which is converted into acetylcholine. A study at Louisiana State University in Baton Rouge shows that starting the day with choline-rich eggs gives a person 20 percent of the daily recommended amount of choline and can reduce hunger, boost energy, and spur the body to burn 83 percent more belly fat. Studies at MIT prove an increase in both choline and acetylcholine in the brains of animals after just one lecithin meal. Supplemental choline has even shown effectiveness in treating Alzheimer's disease.

In addition to low dietary intake of choline itself, low intake of other nutrients (like B vitamins and amino acids) can result in a choline deficiency. Liver problems, including cirrhosis, are common contributing factors to choline deficiency. Certain procedures, such as bypass surgery and kidney transplants, are also direct causes of a choline deficiency.

## Choline, Alzheimer's, and Nutrition

Increased fat oxidation is shown to be an early cause of Alzheimer's disease. Liquid vegetable oils (the polyunsaturated oils) are highly prone to oxidation and rancidity, and it is now well known that in the form of trans-fatty acids (through the process of hydrogenation), they are extremely toxic. These oils are found in packaged foods, including frozen pizzas, prepackaged granola bars, cookies, crackers … you name it! They are in everything. If that isn't scary enough, they are adding TBHQ (tert-Butylhydroquinone) to many of these trans fats. TBHQ is a petrol-derived compound similar to butane (think "lighter fluid" … gross!). And what is this doing to our cells and brain? One gram of TBHQ is found to produce nausea, vomiting, ringing in the ears, delirium, a sense of suffocation, and collapse; five grams is known to kill.

Coconut oil, by contrast, is highly saturated; in its natural unrefined form, it has a shelf life of more than two years and is not prone to oxidation.

Brain tissue is very rich in complex forms of fats. An experiment in which pregnant mice were given diets containing either coconut oil or unsaturated oil showed that brain development was superior in the young mice whose mothers ate coconut oil. Coconut oil supports thyroid function, and our thyroid governs brain development.

Recent research on Alzheimer's has begun to look at a ketogenic diet and its potential benefits. Ketones are a high-energy fuel that nourishes the brain. Our body can produce ketones from stored fat while fasting or in starvation, but they can also be produced by converting medium-chain fatty acids in certain foods. Coconut oil is nature's richest source of these medium-chain triglycerides (MCTs). The high-fat ketogenic diet has been used for years for certain forms of childhood epilepsy, and we are now turning to this diet for Alzheimer's and other diseases as well.

In Alzheimer's disease, certain brain cells have difficulty metabolizing glucose. Without fuel, these precious neurons may begin to die. But now we know there is an alternative energy source for brain cells—ketone bodies. Ketones are a high-energy fuel that nourishes the brain. When you are starving, the body produces ketones naturally. When MCT oil is digested, the liver converts it into ketones. In the first few weeks of life, ketones provide about 25 percent of the energy that newborn babies need to survive.

Non-hydrogenated coconut oil is more than 60 percent MCT oil; this medication derived its MCT oil from the readily available tropical tree.

Alzheimer's patients consuming coconut oil find that it "lifts the fog." Patients taking coconut oil every day see tremendous improvement by the fifth day. Tremors subside, visual disturbances disappear, and patients become more social and interested in people.

While coconut oil is certainly not a cure-all for diseases like Alzheimer's, it does offer hope as nature's most abundant source of MCTs and as an easily convertible fuel source for ketones. People suffering from Alzheimer's should immediately start avoiding polyunsaturated forms of oil ,such as soy and corn oils, especially if the oils are hydrogenated and in the form of trans-fatty acids. A good quality virgin coconut oil should be added to the diet.

The rise in Alzheimer's started after World War II, when there was a rise in industrial vegetable oils. Alzheimer's is not a common disease in tropical cultures where coconut oil and saturated fats are traditionally consumed. Again, it comes down to our brilliant Mother Nature. She knows best. I laugh when people are chowing down on Wheat Thins and claiming, "Oh, you don't want to eat too much coconut oil. That stuff is bad for you." Why? Because of the saturated fat? Yet little do they know, the chemically made "food" they are consuming is doing more harm to their waistline and brain than anything Mother Nature has created for us. It's also important to note that the MCTs in coconut oil cause an increase in phospholipid levels in the brain (which promotes healthy cognitive function), yet does not raise cholesterol concentrations in the parietal cortex.

In 2008, a study in the American *Journal of Clinical Nutrition* compared the use of Coconut oil (MCTs) and olive oil as part of a weight loss diet in a group of people at risk for metabolic syndrome. 31 men and women participated in this 4 month study. They were all overweight and consumed about 12% of their calories from either MCTs or olive oil. At the end of the trial, the scientists concluded that, "MCT oil can be incorporated into a weight loss program without fear of adversely affecting our waist line." Another 2008 experiment found that MCTs can actually improve "cardiac dysfunction" for those with high blood pressure.

## Increase Your Acetylcholine Levels

- Adding MCTs (coconut oil) to your diet helps age-related cognitive decline.

- Increase omega-3 fatty acids, which help in the parietal cortex of the brain (the part of the brain that is severely impacted by Alzheimer's disease).

- Eat any of the following:
  - Grass fed beef
  - Chicken or beef liver
  - Yolks of eggs
  - Pork
  - Sardines and salmon,
  - Shrimp
  - Pine nuts, almonds, hazelnuts, and macadamia nuts
  - Broccoli
  - Brussels sprouts
  - Cucumber, zucchini, and spinach
  - Cheese (if not dairy sensitive)

## Supplements for Acetylcholine

Frankly, the best way to increase your acetylcholine is through supplements. There are some fantastic supplements available. Take these supplements 30 minutes before eating.

CHOLINE (200–3000 mg) Improves physical performance over an extended period of time, thus burning more calories.

ACETYL-L-CARNITINE (500–5000 mg) Aids in fat burning, and improves athletic performance and memory function.

OMEGA-3 (1000–3000 mg) Facilitates fat loss, decreases appetite, increases athletic performance, and enhances brain waves.

CLA (1–6 g) Facilitates fat loss.

PROBIOTICS (1 billion per day) Acidophilus and bifidobacteria balance brain chemistry.

MANGANESE (1–5 mg) A mineral that preserves acetylcholine.

## DOPAMINE: INCREASE METABOLISM

Dopamine regulates activity in the frontal lobe, the area of the brain that controls communication, motivation, and the ability to experience pleasure. Deficits of this chemical have been linked to psychological symptoms like social anxiety, self-criticism, procrastination, and difficulty maintaining relationships. Once deficiencies are corrected, people often feel more energetic, sociable, and confident. Increased dopamine also increases the perception of our senses, as though it is turning up the volume in all of our senses (taste, vision, hearing, smell, and touch).

Dopamine assists cells in converting food and stored fat into usable fuel for the brain. Low levels of dopamine zaps energy and slows metabolism to a halt, causing people to gain a lot of weight very quickly. In fact, research in the scientific journal *Synapse* suggests that women with this deficiency are on average at least 20 percent heavier than their high-dopamine counterparts.

ADD is a symptom of a dopamine deficiency. Becoming quickly bored with routine and having a hard time focusing are classic symptoms. People with dopamine deficiencies tend to start a lot of things, yet don't finish them. They work on a lot of different things at once. In an ADHD child, low levels of dopamine don't allow the child to focus or attend to anything in the environment, making them look very physically hyperactive due to their lack of focus.

A sluggish mind and fatigue are signs you need more dopamine. Low dopamine levels can cause depression, loss of motor control, loss of satisfaction, addictions, cravings, compulsions, low sex drive, and poor attention and focus.

Normally, when a signal needs to travel through the brain, neurons release dopamine to transport the signal across the gap, or synapse, between neurons. A kind of protein pump called a transporter recycles dopamine back to the neurons to prepare for the next burst of signal. Regulating dopamine plays a vital role in our mental and physical health. Neurons containing dopamine are clustered in the midbrain in an area called the substantia nigra. In Parkinson's disease, the dopamine-transmitting neurons in this area die. As a result, the brains of people with Parkinson's disease contain almost no dopamine.

On the other end of the dopamine spectrum, as dopamine levels in the brain begin to rise, we become excited and energized. If it gets too high, which usually happens with drug addictions, then the body becomes overstimulated by our environment, becoming guarded and suspicious. With low levels of dopamine, we can't focus, while with high levels of dopamine, our focus becomes so intense to the point of focusing on everything as though it were directly related to our situation.

Dopamine is associated with addictions. Nicotine, ecstasy, cocaine, and other substances produce a feeling of euphoria by increasing dopamine levels in the brain to an unhealthy level. Too much of these substances make us feel "wired," overstimulated, and unable to determine what's important and what is not.

- Do you often feel depressed, flat, bored, and apathetic?
- Are you low on physical or mental energy?
- Do you feel tired a lot and have to push yourself to exercise?
- Is your drive, enthusiasm, and motivation on the low side?
- Do you have difficulty focusing or concentrating?
- Are you easily chilled? Do you have cold hands or feet?

- Do you tend to put on weight too easily?
- Do you feel the need to get more alert and motivated by consuming a lot of coffee or other "uppers" like sugar, diet soda, ephedra, or even cocaine?

If you answered "yes" to many of the questions above, I recommend that you start taking baby steps to remove foods from your diet that deplete dopamine and start adding foods that boost it. Be aware that dopamine levels typically change very slowly.

Foods that deplete dopamine are sugar, carbohydrates, and high glycemic foods, which include cakes, corn, crackers, chips, pasta, pastries, potatoes, puddings, white breads, and rice. But did I really need to tell you these are bad?

Foods containing phenylalanine reduce fatigue and relieve pain. Foods high in tyrosine also help build more dopamine in your brain. Foods high in phenylalanine and tyrosine include basil, dill, rosemary, mustard seeds, poppy seeds, cinnamon, ginger, peppermint, chicken, grass-fed beef and pork, eggs, and wild game.

## Steps to Increase Dopamine:

1. Eat a keto breakfast instead of a high-sugar breakfast so you no longer need to pack a granola bar, which has as much sugar as a candy bar and will lower dopamine levels. The high-fat and moderate protein of a keto breakfast will keep you full until lunch or late afternoon. Studies in the journal *Metabolism* find that these keto foods can decrease food intake by 11 percent, plus improve mental and physical energy and spur the body to burn more fat.

2. Add in herbs high in tyrosine. I hide fresh herbs in my meatloaf, meatballs, chili, sauces ... all of my cooking. Choose fresh organic herbs.

3. Eliminate your intake of sugar and trans fats. Not only will these products reduce dopamine levels in your bloodstream, but trans fats

will clog your arteries and increase your risk of heart disease. You can still enjoy your favorite foods, but cut out as much sugar as possible and substitute coconut oil in your food preparation.

4. Switch to a decaffeinated Americano in place of your coffee. An Americano is espresso with extra water. Decaf espresso has less caffeine than decaf coffee and it tastes much better than decaf coffee. Caffeine boosts the neurotransmitters in the brain and increases dopamine and serotonin temporarily, but after the spike, dopamine levels sink. People who suffer from depression should avoid caffeinated coffee.

5. Cut out alcohol. Alcohol limits neurotransmitter function and creates a false sense of security that the user comes to depend upon.

6. Supplement your diet with foods rich in antioxidants. Free radicals lower dopamine levels in the body, and antioxidants eliminate free radicals. Herbs and spices are my choices to get high doses of antioxidants, not fruits. If you are eating a keto-adapted diet, the need for antioxidants is reduced, as noted earlier.

7. Add in natural amino acid supplements to get a dopamine boost. Available at health food stores or online, these products offer a concentrated dose of the amino acids naturally found in a healthy brain.

## Supplements to Boost Dopamine

TYROSINE (500–4000 mg) Stimulates the body to burn adipose tissue and increases hormones that produce satiety.

PHENYLALANINE (500–1000 mg twice daily, divided into three doses on empty stomach) The amino acids tyrosine and phenylalanine, which are compounds used by the brain to produce dopamine, are the brain's source of power and energy.

L-GLUTAMINE (3 g) Helps convert amino acids into brain neurotransmitters and is involved in preventing cravings for carbohydrates, drugs and alcohol, energy levels, and mood.

CHROMIUM (100–1000 mcg) Stabilizes blood sugar levels and helps reduce cravings.

B VITAMINS (10–500 mg) Take this in the morning to increase energy.

OMEGA-3(EPA/DHA) (1000–3000 mg) Take this 3 times a day at each meal. High levels increase fat loss and reduce appetite.

MAGNESIUM Glycinate (400–1000 mg) Take this in the evening to help with sleep. It also reduces chocolate cravings.

VITAMIN-D (5000 IU with food if your levels are below 50) Vitamin D in the adrenal gland regulates tyrosine hydroxylase, the rate limiting enzyme necessary for the production of dopamine, epinephrine and norepinephrine.

SAME (400–1600 mg) Taken in the morning, it is the first metabolite of the essential amino acid, L-methionine.

PROBIOTICS (1 billion per day) Acidophilus and bifidobacteria balance brain chemistry.

## SLEEP

Do you think that getting away with only five, six, or seven hours of sleep is just fine? Sleep is our bodies' way of recharging our hormones, cells, and neurotransmitters for the next round of daily stressors. It is the period in which we lower the energy and stress levels expelled each day, we balance out thyroid hormone, our muscles and soft tissues repair and revitalize, and our mind is able to process memories and things we have learned for the day. Having one day of sleep deprivation is not fatal, but it will cause a decrease in emotional, physical, and overall function. Overtime, these negative changes become bigger concerns such as weight gain, thyroid disorders, high blood pressure, and a decrease in the immune system.

Without a restful night's sleep, vicious cycles can begin leading to fatigue, performance, and mood disruptions. Quality sleep will help with balancing your brain, hormones, and cravings and will get you back to your happy, natural rhythm.

My clients love when I give them the assignment of getting more sleep. Some lose 4 pounds just by adding a few hours of sleep a night, without changing their diet. One of my heavier clients lost 17 pounds in six days just by adding natural sleep supplements. This helped her increase her sleep from two hours a night to seven hours. According to the National Sleep Foundation, most people need at least eight hours of high-quality sleep every night. I say "high-quality" because a night brought on by Tylenol PM or alcohol is not quality sleep. Quality sleep is when our bodies get into the rapid eye movement state (also called REM). REM sleep is a peak time for growth and repair, and if we don't get enough, our health and metabolism will suffer.

Sleep deprivation impairs our ability to metabolize carbohydrates and it increases our stress hormones. This can lead to high blood sugar, high insulin levels, unbalanced neurotransmitters, and weight gain. If you are staying awake to get more things done, to surf the Internet, or to watch TV, you are not alone. Our society seems to reward people for working more and sleeping less. The pharmaceutical industry encourages this dysfunctional sleep pattern by offering drugs that help you fall asleep and drugs that help you wake up. Now is the time for us to start making an effort to get more sleep. Chronic sleep deprivation can have a variety of effects on the metabolism and overall health. The following are some ways in which sleep deprivation affects our bodies:

- Interferes with the body's ability to metabolize carbohydrates and causes high levels of glucose in the blood. This leads to higher insulin levels. Insulin is not only toxic, but it is our "fat-storing" hormone.

- Decreases serotonin

- Decreases leptin production, which causes an intense desire for carbohydrates.

- Reduces human growth hormone production, which is our "fat-burning" hormone

- Causes imbalances in our neurotransmitters and increases depression and anxiety
- Increases risk of diabetes
- Increases blood pressure
- Increases risk of heart disease
- Increases obesity
- Increases rates of breast cancer
- Increases memory loss

Sleep is a complex neurological chain of events. Many neurotransmitters and hormones are necessary at certain levels to achieve sleep, and just as many can prevent us from attaining a good night's sleep.

## Why Sleep:

1. Mood. Sleep loss results in a decrease in our neurotransmitters, causing depression, irritability, impatience, an inability to focus, and anxiety. Too little sleep can also leave you too tired to do the things you enjoy in life.

2. Metabolism and weight. Chronic sleep deprivation causes weight gain by altering the levels of hormones that affect our appetite and the way we process and store carbohydrates. Less sleep means a decrease in thyroid output, an increase in the ghrelin hormone (hunger hormone), and an decrease in human growth hormone (fat-burning hormone).

3. Cardiovascular health. Serious sleep disorders have been linked to hypertension, increased stress hormone levels (i.e., cortisol … think belly fat), and an irregular heartbeat.

4. Disease. A lack of sleep decreases the functions of our immune system, including the activity of the body's killer cells. Adequate sleep helps fight cancer.

5. Learning and memory. Sleep allows the brain to accept new information to memory through a process called memory consolidation.

Nerve-signaling chemicals called neurotransmitters control whether we are asleep or awake by acting on different groups of nerve cells, or neurons, in the brain. Neurons in the brain stem, which connects the brain with the spinal cord, produce neurotransmitters such as serotonin and norepinephrine that keep some parts of the brain active while we are awake. Other neurons at the base of the brain begin signaling when we fall asleep. These neurons appear to "switch off" the signals that keep us awake. Research also suggests that a chemical called adenosine builds up in our blood while we are awake and causes drowsiness. This chemical gradually breaks down while we sleep.

In a healthy body, we pass through five phases of sleep: stages 1, 2, 3, 4, and REM (rapid eye movement) sleep. These phases happen in a cycle, starting at stage 1 and finishing in REM sleep; the cycle then starts over again with stage 1. We spend around 50 percent of our total sleep time in stage 2 sleep, about 20 percent in REM sleep, and the remaining 30 percent in the other stages. Babies spend about half of their sleep time in REM sleep.

During stage 1 (light sleep), we drift in and out of sleep and can be awakened easily. Our eyes move very slowly and our muscle activity slows. People awakened from stage 1 sleep often remember pieces of visual images or experience sudden muscle contractions called hypnic myoclonia. This is often followed by a sensation of falling. In stage 2 sleep, our eye movements stop and our brain waves become slower, with small bursts of rapid waves called sleep spindles. In stage 3, very slow brain waves called delta waves start to emerge, combined with shorter, faster waves. By stage 4, the brain produces delta waves almost exclusively. It is very difficult to wake someone in stages 3 and 4, which are known as deep sleep. There is no eye movement or muscle activity. People awakened during deep sleep feel groggy and disoriented. Children may experience sleepwalking, bed-wetting, or night terrors during deep sleep.

When we switch into REM sleep, our breathing becomes more rapid, irregular, and shallow; our eyes move rapidly in different directions; and our limbs become momentarily paralyzed. Our heart rate increases, our blood pressure rises, and males develop erections. When people awaken during REM sleep, they often remember dreams. The first REM sleep period usually occurs about 70 to 90 minutes after we fall asleep. People lose some ability to regulate body temperature during REM, so abnormally hot or cold temperatures in the environment can disrupt this stage of sleep. If our REM sleep is disrupted one night, our bodies don't follow the normal sleep cycle progression the next time we doze off. Instead, we often slip directly into REM sleep and go through extended periods of REM until we "catch up" on this stage of sleep.

Since sleep and wakefulness are influenced by different neurotransmitter signals in the brain, everything we consume, from foods to medicines, changes the balance of these signals and affects how well we sleep. Caffeine found in chocolate, coffee, tea, and drugs such as diet pills or decongestants stimulates parts of the brain and can cause insomnia, the inability to sleep. Most antidepressants suppress REM sleep, which then causes weight gain, cravings, and more mood disorders. Heavy smokers often sleep very lightly and have reduced amounts of REM sleep. They also tend to wake up after three or four hours of sleep due to nicotine withdrawal, craving a dopamine spike. Many people who suffer from insomnia try to solve the problem with alcohol (the so-called "night cap"). While alcohol helps people fall into light sleep, it also robs them of REM and the deeper, more restorative stages of sleep. By keeping them in the lighter stages of sleep, never balancing their brain, alcohol creates a snowball effect for the next day where the brain craves alcohol.

Deep sleep coincides with the release of the human growth hormone, which is our fat-burning hormone. Many of the body's cells also show increased production and reduced breakdown of proteins during deep sleep. Since proteins are the building blocks needed for cell growth and for the repair of damage from factors like stress, deep sleep is truly "beauty sleep." Activity in the parts of the brain that control emotions, decision-making processes, and social interactions is drastically reduced during deep sleep, showing that this type of sleep helps people maintain optimal emotional and social functioning while they are awake.

Neurons that control sleep interact closely with the immune system. As anyone who has had the flu knows, infectious diseases tend to make us feel sleepy. This happens because cytokines, the chemicals our immune systems produce while fighting an infection, are powerful sleep-inducing chemicals. Sleep helps the body conserve energy and other resources that the immune system needs to attack viruses and illnesses.

## Sleep and Serotonin

Serotonin levels are highest in the brain stem when you are awake and active and are almost completely absent when we enter REM sleep, the deepest stage of sleep. During sleep, the body's level of melatonin rises sharply. The production of melatonin is dependent on its synthesis in the pineal gland, which is powered by serotonin. While light increases the production of serotonin, darkness spurs on the synthesis of melatonin. Paired together, these two neurotransmitters are key to maintaining the sleep cycle. We need a good balance of serotonin and melatonin to keep us from burning out. If we skimp on sleep and keep our serotonin high, we will wear out our brain's production of serotonin, causing intense cravings and mood disorders.

Anything that disrupts the rhythm of serotonin and melatonin production will disturb the natural sleep cycle. When you suffer from jet lag, for instance, your serotonin production cycle follows that of your home time zone and has trouble getting on track. During the winter, when sunlight inadequately triggers the production of serotonin, sleep cycles can also be interrupted.

One cause of poor sleep is sleep apnea, a condition that can sometimes be caused by a decline in serotonin. The nerves that control breathing need serotonin in order to do their job. A malfunctioning serotonin system deprives the body of a sufficient supply of this neurotransmitter, resulting in sleep apnea. It has been found that in these apnea cases, the use of a serotonin precursor, such as 5-HTP, can alleviate sleep apnea. Doctors who promote the use of 5-HTP recommend that apnea patients take 100 to 300 mg of it before going to bed. In most cases, the outcome is more restful sleep with less awakenings, and increased focus and productivity the next day. Of course, you should check with your doctor before taking 5-HTP.

## Sleep and GABA

Sleep problems and anxiety disorders can also result from problems with GABA, which helps neutralize the effects of glutamate, a brain chemical that causes excitement. GABA is the most plentiful of the inhibitory neurotransmitters of the brain; it stabilizes the brain by preventing an overexcited mode and instead delivers a calming effect to the brain. When there is too little GABA, it causes those racing thoughts that characterize anxiety and keep you up at night.

Specifically, GABA deficiencies interfere with the most important stage of sleep, the "deep" delta sleep that usually begins within 45 minutes after bedtime. Studies show that people with depression, anxiety, and other mood disorders are usually deficient in delta sleep. The longer GABA-related sleep problems continue, the greater the risk to your brain health. One in three people with recurrent insomnia has some type of psychiatric disorder, and 25% have anxiety, nearly three times the rate of those whose insomnia has been treated.

Higher levels of human growth hormone, or HGH, are caused by the stimulating effect GABA has on the anterior pituitary. The pituitary is the main endocrine gland controlling all hormonal functions of the body, the human growth hormone being the main one. HGH, which seems to be in sparse supply after the age of 40, is thought to be the reason for interrupted sleep cycles and sleep disruptions.

There have been several hundred clinical studies on how GABA neurotransmitters elevate growth hormone levels, hormones that have an effect on sleep cycles. According to a study performed at the University of Milan in Italy, HGH levels were significantly increased by GABA administration. This in turn has a positive effect on functions such as sleep cycles, average body temperatures, and pituitary gland action.

It has been determined that GABA has the ability to elevate growth hormone levels and fat burning capabilities. HGH is naturally released within ninety minutes of falling asleep. So, whether taking GABA for fat loss or to help induce sleep with improved sleep cycles, this supplement should be taken immediately before bedtime. GABA promotes quality sleep.

GABA levels have been found to be lower in people with disorders such as multiple sclerosis and other movement disorders. People with panic anxiety, depression, alcoholism, and bipolar disorders have low GABA levels. Diet, prolonged stress, and genetics have much to do with GABA deficiencies. The side effects of GABA supplements are little to none. Sleepiness is one possible side effect, which is why GABA neurotransmitters will productively induce sleep and will benefit those who experience interrupted sleep cycles.

## Sleep and Dopamine

Just one night without sleep can increase the amount of the chemical dopamine in the human brain. Drugs that increase dopamine, like amphetamines, promote wakefulness; the following research explains how the brain helps people stay awake despite feeling the urge to sleep. Scientists have found that in healthy participants, sleep deprivation increased dopamine in two brain structures: the striatum, which is involved in motivation and reward, and the thalamus, which is involved in alertness. They also found that the amount of dopamine in the brain correlated with feelings of fatigue and impaired performance of cognitive tasks. The concurrent decline in cognitive performance, which is associated with increases in dopamine, suggests that the adaptation is not sufficient to overcome the cognitive deterioration induced by sleep deprivation, and may even contribute to it.

Dopamine plays a critical role in regulating sleep and brain activity associated with dreaming. When dopamine levels are dramatically reduced, we can no longer sleep. Patients suffering from Parkinson's disease often suffer from sleep disorders. Research may lead to the development of new diagnostic tools for the early detection of Parkinson's disease (based on the sleep disturbances that are often associated with motor symptoms of the disease). Parkinson's disease occurs when the brain cells, or neurons, that normally produce dopamine die or become impaired. Once 60 to 70 percent of the neurons are knocked out of commission, the jerky movements and fixed facial expressions that are characteristic of Parkinson's appear.

## Restless Legs Syndrome

Restless legs syndrome (RLS) is a disorder that causes unpleasant tingling, jerking, or crawling sensations in the legs and feet and causes an urge to frequently move these limbs for relief. It is emerging as one of the most common sleep disorders, especially among older people. This disorder, which affects as many as 12 million Americans, leads to constant leg movement during the day and insomnia at night. Severe RLS is most common in elderly people, though symptoms may develop at any age. In some cases, it may be linked to other conditions such as pregnancy, anemia, or diabetes.

RLS often can be relieved by drugs that affect the neurotransmitter dopamine, a fact that suggests that dopamine abnormalities underlie these disorders' symptoms. Taking DL-phenylalanine and L-tyrosine can help increase dopamine production (see chapter 5 on supplements for more information). RLS is also a sign of a magnesium deficiency. I suggest taking 400–800 mg of magnesium glycinate 30 minutes before bed. If your restless leg does not go away with L-tyrosine and magnesium, then the cause is most likely low iron. I do not recommend taking iron unless you know your iron levels. I suggest getting a ferritin test to properly test iron levels.

## Lack of Sleep and Hormones

Many studies make a link between sleep and the hormones that manipulate our eating behavior (ghrelin and leptin). Have you ever experienced a sleepless night followed by a day where no matter what you ate, you never felt satisfied? This is the outcome when leptin and ghrelin get out of balance. Leptin and ghrelin work like a "checks and balances" system that manages hunger and fullness. Ghrelin, produced in the stomach, increases appetite, while leptin, produced in fat cells, sends a message to our brain when we are full. A lack of sleep causes ghrelin levels to increase and your leptin levels to decrease. This imbalance causes us to intensely crave food and never feel full. The worst part is that we don't crave broccoli ... we crave high-calorie sweets and starchy foods. Over time, this imbalance can easily lead to long-term weight gain.

When summer approaches, people often think they are going to lose weight because we are more active in the summer. But do you lose weight? Or do you gain weight? Many people actually gain weight in the summer, and one main reason is that they skimp on sleep. It is easy to get 8 to10 hours of sleep when it gets dark out at 4:30 p.m. in January, but who wants to go to bed when it is still light out? Not me! I work with a lot of gastric bypass patients, and in the past, we uses to think that they had sleep apnea after they gained weight; now, we know that lack of sleep = leptin resistance = not getting the sense of feeling full = overeating = weight gain! Bad, bad, bad.

In a Chicago study, doctors analyzed leptin and ghrelin levels in twelve fit men. They started by charting their normal levels of appetite and hunger. The men were assigned two days of sleep deprivation followed by two days of limitless sleep. Doctors supervised hormone levels, appetite, and activity level. The men had considerable changes. When sleep was restricted, leptin levels went down and ghrelin levels went up. As expected, the men's appetite also increased: the desire for high-carbohydrate and high-calorie foods increased by a shocking 45 percent. These cravings also occurred because of the imbalance of serotonin.

A Stanford study found an interesting significance of the leptin–ghrelin effect. Researchers studied 1,000 volunteers that reported the number of hours they slept each night. The doctors then analyzed the volunteers' levels of ghrelin and leptin and their weight. The numbers show that the volunteers who slept less than eight hours a night not only had lower levels of leptin and higher levels of ghrelin, but also had higher levels of body fat. A link was made when researchers discovered that the volunteers' levels of body fat correlated with their sleep patterns. Those who slept the fewest hours per night weighed the most.

Don't throw your walking shoes away just because this is an easier way to lose weight. Studies also show the relationship is not as obvious as it seems. An interesting problem called "obstructive sleep apnea" is something that most people have without knowing it. This causes an imbalance in our hormone levels. People with sleep apnea stop breathing for up to a minute sometimes hundreds of times throughout the night. This condition is mysterious because the true cause of the problem is unknown. Some doctors believe that a physical deformity inside the throat causes soft tissue to collapse. This briefly pinches the air passages during the night, causing a disruption in breathing and a tendency to snore. So even though you are unconscious for eight hours, the disrupted breathing stops you from getting quality sleep. Eight hours of disrupted sleep can leave you feeling like you had only four or five hours of sleep. One symptom of sleep apnea is that you wake up feeling tired, even though you might have gone to bed early. People who suffer from sleep apnea are more likely to be overweight. The confusing part is that doctors find people with sleep apnea have oddly high levels of leptin, the hormone that turns off hunger. Another interesting fact is that when patients' apnea is treated, leptin levels drop, an event that somehow helps them to lose weight. Confused? Me, too.

As it turns out, the level of leptin in our bodies doesn't matter as much as our response to it. I began to understand this concept when researchers examined people who are "insulin resistant"; these people have plenty of insulin, but their bodies can't recognize it because they became desensitized. In the case of people with apnea, their bodies are resistant to the "fullness" signal that leptin sends to the brain. Their bodies are trying to tell them to stop eating, but their brains aren't getting the message. Experts believe that our exercise patterns, eating habits, stress levels, and genetics all control the production and response of leptin and ghrelin.

Sleeping less can also affect changes in our basal metabolic rate (the number of calories you burn when you rest). When you are sleeping, your body produces human growth hormone, the stuff celebrities are now injecting in themselves to look and feel young. Human growth hormone helps preserve our muscle and keeps our metabolism firing at night. So an inadequate amount of sleep will keep this highly desired hormone from kicking in. Another thing to remember is that our human growth hormone doesn't kick in if we eat three hours before bed.

A lack of sleep increases the release of the stress hormone (cortisol), stimulates hunger, and tells us to hold onto those carbohydrates in our belly fat. A lack of sleep can also slow our thyroid hormones, which have a huge impact on our metabolism.

When you get a good night's rest, your body has adequate time to repair and rejuvenate. Adults need between seven and nine hours of quality sleep per night for optimal health. Children and teenagers require even more. Some people just don't have enough time in the day to get enough sleep, and millions of Americans chronically experience trouble with falling asleep, waking in the night, or both. Here are some tips I use to help me get 8 hours of quality sleep:

- Avoid sugar and foods high in carbohydrates like popcorn, chips, and crackers. It causes low quality sleep and can cause you to wake up in the middle of the night with low blood sugar. When your blood sugar gets too high, it crashes down, causing disturbed sleep. A keto-adapted diet keeps your blood sugar nice and even all night long.

- Follow a regular sleep schedule by going to bed and rising at the same time.

- Before bed, do something to relax your muscles and your mind (stretching, yoga, or deep breathing exercises).

- Reduce or eliminate caffeine (chocolate has caffeine, so beware).

- Turn off the TV and computer and darken your bedroom with heavy drapes.

- Turn the heat down. I often sleep with the windows open even in the winter; I sleep the best at about 57 degrees.

- Add natural supplements to your diet.

**PROGESTERONE, SLEEP AND ANXIETY:** If you fall asleep easily, but tend to wake up at 3 or 4 a.m. wide awake, the cause is most likely low progesterone. This can happen to women who are menopausal and to those not in menopause. I have seen estrogen dominance in 20-year-olds. Low progesterone causes anxiety and an inability to sleep. I suggest adding in a pure progesterone cream on your wrist at night.

If these healthy habits don't solve your insomnia, millions of Americans, including myself, take 400 to 800 mg of magnesium glycinate at bedtime. This mineral is a natural muscle relaxant and can help calm anxiety, both things that help with sleep. Dr. Carolyn Dean's *The Magnesium Miracle* is an amazing book that explains the effects of magnesium in detail. If taking this supplement does not work for you, then it is time to contact a health professional or nutritionist to inquire about progesterone cream, 5-HTP, or melatonin. These are effective and natural ways to improve sleep. We are all pressed for time in our lives, but I encourage you to find eight hours for sleep to maximize energy, mood, mental focus, and metabolism. It is the easiest way to maximize our health, with no painful exercises required.

# SUPPLEMENTING OUR BRAIN

*Hey all! I waited to have a full three months of success maintaining my weight because in all honesty, that has never happened for me after losing weight. I have experience with WW [Weight Watchers] and exercising my brains out, and any time I met my goal weight then backed off my regimen, I gained weight back. Super frustrating. I have always been an active person that enjoys fitness, but I have also continually weighed the heaviest healthiest weight for my height. A year after having my third baby, at my heaviest weight, and age 40, I started working with Maria. Now I have been in the middle of my healthy weight range and am wearing the same size jeans I did in high school and college. That is amazing for a 41-year-old woman who has worn two sizes larger for the last twelve years.*

*I was skeptical in the beginning about everything, especially the supplements. I decided that since she was only asking me to take them until I healed my body, it was worth the investment. I have to admit I did accumulate some debt changing over my entire pantry and purchasing all the recommended supplements. At about three months, I decided I wasn't going to repurchase an expensive supplement, but I was super crabby and short with my kids and decided I should get one more bottle because I just knew going off the supplement was the reason for feeling so edgy. Sure enough, after a few days back on the supplement, I was calmer and less irritable. After completing that bottle it had been six months and though I was afraid to not take it, I didn't have any issues.*

*Healed? I think so. Maria has also helped me identify a health issue the doctors kept labeling as heart burn. As it turns out, I had a bit more than a sensitivity to dairy. Too much dairy and I get a burning in my intestines that I really feel in the late hours of night or early morning. No dairy, no burning. I also learned that when I indulge in dairy, my skin breaks out. I suffered from adult acne until I ate the Maria way. Because of my burning tummy issues, I also went dairy free for four months and had the most beautiful skin. Now I know the secret to beautiful skin for me.*

*I got really lazy this month. I haven't taken supplements, lifted, or done yoga. I feel like crap, but I haven't gained weight. I am still in my comfortable three-pound range I like, but I know I won't be happy unless I take care of myself, like Maria recommends. My biggest issue before working with Maria was not sleeping well. And that is what is most challenging: not taking my supplements. I have been walking our six-month-old puppy 3 to 4 days a week for a half hour to hour, so I know it's not a lack of physical activity.*

*This is it. My honest testimony of my experience working Maria. I did it all. I put it to the test and now I know what is good for me, what makes me feel good. I will faithfully take supplements upon awaking, some during meals, and always my bedtime ones. I will not eat three hours before sleeping. I will attempt to get 7.5 to 8 hours of sleep. I will lift or go to yoga at least twice a week. The food stuff is easy; I'm now going on nine months of (re)learning to cook and bake. I couldn't do it without Maria's recipe books.*

*In summation, I lost 30 pounds, my acne went away, my stomach pain went away, my mood lifted, I am a better Mommy and better person, my husband enjoys this improved version of me, and I have great hope for a long, happy life.*

*Oh, and my numbers from my annual physical in June were perfect. Thank you, Maria!*

## PROBIOTICS: THE "GUT–BRAIN" CONNECTION

Probiotics are beneficial bacteria that help keep your digestive system healthy. The majority of my clients have malfunctioning digestive systems for a variety of reasons. Our typical "Western" eating habits and stress can all negatively impact the good bacteria in our gut. Probiotics are helpful micro-organisms that live in our intestinal tract. In a healthy body, good bacteria make up most of the intestines' micro-flora and protect digestive health. If you primarily have good bacteria, your immune system will function optimally and will help you extract essential nutrients in the foods you eat. Remember, in order to feed our cells, we need to absorb the nutrients from our food, otherwise our brain will keep telling us to eat until the cells are fed.

If you suffer from one or more of the problems listed below, it is quite likely that taking a probiotic supplement can help you get your "system" back on the right track. The following are the most common warning signs of a bacterial imbalance:

1.  Allergies and food sensitivities
2.  Difficulty losing weight, sugar or carbohydrate cravings
3.  Frequent fatigue, poor concentration
4.  Frequent constipation or diarrhea
5.  Faulty digestion, acid reflux, and other gut disorders
6.  Sleeping poorly, night sweats
7.  Painful joint inflammation, stiffness
8.  Bad breath, gum disease, and dental problems
9.  Frequent colds, flu, or infections
10. Chronic yeast problems
11. Acne, eczema, and foot fungus
12. Extreme menstrual or menopausal symptoms

There are many stresses and factors that can kill your "friendly bacteria" every day. The following is a summary of some of the most common good bacteria killers:

1.  Antibiotics
2.  Birth control pills
3.  Steroidal and hormonal drugs
4.  Fluoride (added to toothpaste and sometimes to drinking water)
5.  Chlorine (a chemical added to water to kill bacteria — it kills your friendly bacteria, too)
6.  Laxatives and diarrhea

7. Coffee, soda, and some teas

8. Synthetic vitamins (manufactured vitamin supplements)

9. Radiation (including TVs and cell phones)

10. Stress

11. Preservatives

12. Additives (colorings, flavorings, and chemicals in processed foods)

13. Pesticides (choose organic fruit and veggies to avoid this!)

14. Fertilizers (choose organic fruit and veggies to avoid this!)

## Probiotics and Brain Health

Our moods are directly correlated to the intestinal flora of our gut. The nervous system actually begins in the gut and travels to the brain; in the past, it was believed the nervous system ran the other way. This is why what we put in our stomach is so essential to our mental health. Having healthy intestinal flora ,which you can achieve with probiotics and fermented foods, increases our moods and decreases our cravings.

"Good bacteria," taken in pill or powder form, help maintain healthy gut flora that are beneficial to our general health. Countless studies have shown them to perform a wide variety of healthy functions, including improving digestion and regularity and improving the function of the immune system. But there is new groundbreaking news that having healthy bacteria has significant effects on the body, specifically on the feel-good neurotransmitter L-tryptophan. Probiotics truly have a role to play in the management of brain disorders like anxiety and depression.

Probiotics "crowd out" the more toxic stomach bacteria linked to depression and other mood disorders. Bifidobacteria increase levels of tryptophan in the brain, which is a chemical that helps people "feel better." Patients taking probiotics also show a marked improvement in their digestion, experience less bloating and gas, and have a reduction in inflammation. People taking probiotics feel calmer, sleep better, have less anxiety, feel more able to cope with illness, and have fewer heart palpitations.

It has been found that people who are identified as suffering from chronic fatigue syndrome (CFS) who boost "good" bacteria in their guts have extreme relief from pain; they also have a significant decrease in depression and anxiety. People with CFS endure an assortment of symptoms, including constant exhaustion, neuropsychological problems like cognitive dysfunction (a condition that occurs from anomalous functioning of the brain and leads to specific behavioral changes), anxiety, depression, nervousness, worries, and despair and sleeping disorders. Those with CFS also experience gastrointestinal troubles like irritable bowel syndrome (IBS). By simply adding in good bacteria to their diets, people find that many symptoms subside within days.

## Probiotics and Weight Loss

An interesting issue related to the struggle to lose weight is gut bacterial overgrowth. Unfortunately, there is an alarming misconception about bacterial overgrowth in our country. The problem is not only with an overgrowth of bad bacteria, but with too much bacteria in general. Recent studies uncovered the additional functions of bacteria in our bodies. One example demonstrates that bacteria helps us to survive in times of famine by extracting extra calories from our food that would normally have been burned off during normal digestion; instead, these calories are stored as fat. I don't think any of us have to worry about starving to death anytime soon.

Bacterial overgrowth can be a result of antibiotics, other medications, colonics or enemas, colonoscopies, stress, poor diet, overconsumption of yeast, low stomach acid, caffeine, and alcohol. People with poor intestinal flora often suffer from intestinal discomfort, yeast infections, candida, constipation, bloating, and weight gain. Reintroducing probiotics quickly normalizes digestive health, prevents infections, strengthens the immune system, and helps you lose weight.

Treating bacteria overgrowth depends on the severity; adding probiotics and changing your diet will help with mild cases. This sounds easy, but depriving yourself of your favorite foods can be challenging. Stay away from refined sugar and grains; fermented foods like beer, wine, and vinegar (mustards); yeast breads; and dried fruit.

Probiotics are also found in the small intestine where they assist the body in multiple digestive and protective processes, including the absorption of minerals and vitamins and the blocking of yeasts, harmful bacteria, and viruses, such as salmonella, E. coli, candida, and herpes. Probiotics can even neutralize cancer-causing toxins, which are produced by our bodies from nitrates and nitrites contained in processed meats and cigarette smoke.

Many practitioners prescribe probiotics to help obese people lose weight by stimulating their metabolism and killing destructive intestinal micro-organisms that contribute to a larger waistline. Recent studies have shown that helpful bacteria can metabolize complex carbohydrates, such as beans, starches, and difficult-to-digest vegetables, therefore reducing bloating, accumulation of waste, and stomach pains (which are typical when fiber consumption is increased).

If you are struggling with your weight and common gut issues, such as gas, bloating, indigestion, constipation, diarrhea, feeling full yet hungry, and persistent skin problems, you could be under attack by an overgrowth of bacteria. Unless you take action to resolve the overgrowth of bacteria, your body will resist losing even an ounce of fat. The overconsumption of yeast is a major factor in weight gain. Taking a probiotic for weight loss will prevent the pounds from piling on.

The most common probiotic for weight loss found today is called acidophilus and is available in capsule form. These healthy bacteria can prevent digestive problems and are also known to help Crohn's disease sufferers. Probiotics for weight loss also help the thyroid gland, which in turn increases metabolism. This gives people with thyroid problems a much needed boost in shedding excess weight.

Bifidobacteria is another helpful probiotic, found in the large intestine and colon. The main function of bifidobacteria is to inhibit the growth of bad bacteria and to absorb the essential B vitamins. Recent science shows that bifidobacteria also reduce "bad" cholesterol levels. Bifidobacteria is found in mothers' breast milk and is essential for babies' digestion. If your baby is suffering from chronic stomach pains, adding bifidobacteria to a quality formula is extremely helpful.

HEALTH TIP: Food manufacturers quickly jumped on the bandwagon soon after scientists touted how essential good bacteria can be for weight loss. The market became flooded with "stomach-friendly" processed products, mainly yogurts containing "live bacteria." TV advertisements show active, happy, and slim women holding cups of probiotic yogurts. Yes, probiotics can help us lose weight, but not when it is mixed with a plastic container filled with high fructose corn syrup.

Healthy indigenous people from various parts of the world have always included bacteria-rich foods in their daily menu; fermented dairy, vegetables, and even fish and meats were consistently consumed by the lean Inuit, Masai, Maori, Russians, Norwegians, and many other early societies. The healthy bacteria produced trim bodies and superior health.

In order to get more probiotics in your diet, be it for weight loss purposes or to improve intestinal health, you can get them from natural food sources, just as our ancestors did. Fermented vegetables like sauerkraut and kimchi are just a few examples of the vast array of foods containing probiotics. If you aren't a fan of these foods, it is cheap and easy to add a supplemental probiotic. I always take these after I need a round of antibiotics.

If you decide to take a probiotic for weight loss, you should always use the most effective strain of probiotics that create an environment that yeasts cannot survive in. Probiotics for weight loss in capsule form should always be stored in the fridge to prevent them from "dying" and becoming useless.

These probiotics in capsule form can be purchased from most health food stores or from the Internet, but remember that they must be kept cool; ensure the shipping time is not too long and that the storage facilities are adequate.

## B VITAMINS: OUR STRESS VITAMINS

If you are taking a prescription medication, you should start taking a B complex vitamin ASAP! A huge unknown side effect of medications is their ability to deplete B vitamins from our bloodstream. Symptoms of a vitamin B deficiency are linked directly to depression, forgetfulness, vague fears, uneasiness and panic, mood swings, rage, morbid thoughts, hostility, restlessness, apprehension, the constant feeling that something dreadful is going to happen, suspiciousness, instability, anxiety, mental confusion, noise sensitivity, inability to handle stress, loss of concentration, loss of memory, nervousness, weakness, fatigue, light-headedness or dizziness, digestive problems, hypochlorhydria (insufficient stomach acid production), constipation or diarrhea, stomach pains, decreased or increased appetite, a craving for sweets, heart palpitations, chest pains, neuralgia to neuritis, muscular soreness, pain, tingling or achiness, cold hands and feet, heightened sensitivity to touch and/or pain, menstrual complaints, soreness of the mouth, dermatitis, acne, burning or itching eyes, difficulty swallowing, sore throat, hypochondria, headaches, insomnia, and sleep disturbances. Yikes, I'm running to my cabinet to take another dose right now!

Choline is a B vitamin that is the precursor of the neurotransmitter acetylcholine and is essential for optimal memory function. Choline, being water soluble, is absorbed through the blood-brain barrier and protects and nourishes other chemicals that support memory. Choline, along with B12, is necessary for myelin formation.

HEALTH TIP: B12 vitamin deficiencies are common in people over 40 because like many of the B vitamins, it relies upon stomach acid to be absorbed. Unlike the other B vitamins, B12 also needs to bond with something called "intrinsic factor." Those of Scandinavian, English, and Irish descent often lack this "intrinsic factor" (produced by the parietal cells of the stomach). I note age 40 (though it could happen earlier) because as we age our digestion slows and we produce less digestive enzymes and less intrinsic factor, which is why sublingual forms (under the tongue) of B12 are more absorbable.

Inositol, another part of the B complex, is also remarkably effective against depression, panic attacks, and obsessive-compulsive disorder (OCD) in several studies. The effective dose is 12 grams per day for four weeks. Inositol has no side effects and is as effective as prescription drugs.

All of the B vitamins are water soluble, meaning they don't last long in your body and must be replaced. Though water soluble, B12 is stored in the liver and therefore is not washed away like most water soluble vitamins. It may take years to develop a B12 deficiency; however, the resulting neurological effects will be noticed before it can be detected by the usual blood tests. Testing urine levels of methylmalonic acid is the best way of assessing a B12 deficiency. This test will detect a deficiency before the blood levels of B12 will record outside the normal range. A B12 deficiency causes the slow and irreversible progression of nerve damage. New evidence suggests that B12 can be deficient even though destructive anemia is not present. Even in cases where the blood does not indicate it, B12 may be dangerously deficient and can contribute to such problems as mental deterioration, confusion, depression, and other cognitive problems.

The best form of B12 is methylcobalamin. This type seems to reverse nerve damage and has been reported in medical literature to help prevent and reverse peripheral nerve damage in conditions that include multiple sclerosis, diabetes, and nerve damage caused by chemotherapy.

Vegetarians are often deficient in B vitamins as the foods richest in B vitamins are animal products. There are B vitamins found in nutritional yeast and seaweeds, however there is also a great controversy over whether they are the same quality.

Folic acid is part of the B vitamin family as well and can relieve depression better than antidepressants alone, with women in particular benefitting the most.

Few people know that the brain is 60% cholesterol. Perhaps fewer know that lecithin makes up about 30% of the dry weight of the brain. Lecithin contains a lot of choline and contains a vitamin not yet recognized by nutritionists called vitamin J. Vitamin J is pure brain food and is needed for good, healthy nerves. Lecithin also contains phosphatidylserine. It was once thought that once brain cells die, they're gone forever, and that new brain cells cannot be grown. However, more than sixty human studies and over 3000 scientific papers have shown that new brain cells *can* be grown Even Alzheimer's symptoms, such as language deterioration, fatigue, depression, poor judgment, vision, and hearing loss, can be reversed. It's the phosphatidylserine in lecithin that does it. You can add liquid lecithin to salad oils for an extra boost.

The best B vitamins are found in food. If you are taking a B vitamin complex or a daily multi-vitamin, keep this in mind: most vitamins are not helpful. Your body cannot survive on synthetic food, so how is it supposed to survive on synthetic vitamins? Always purchase non-synthetic B vitamins.

## VITAMIN D

Have you ever had your vitamin D levels checked? Did your doctor claim you were in the "normal" range, but didn't give you the number? Call and ask. I fell into the "normal" range, only to find out my number was only 31; optimally, we want to be around 70 (**Note:** above 90 can cause problems too). I was shocked to find out I was only 31 considering I was taking 2000

IU of vitamin D for months and I also am outside a lot, even in winter months. In the July 2007 issue of the *New England Journal of Medicine*, a report was published claiming that the widespread vitamin D deficiency in our population affects as much as one billion people. After discovering my own number, I increased my vitamin D intake to 5000 IU daily — I feel better already!

> **HEALTH TIP: Always take vitamin K2 if you take vitamin D supplements.**

The following are some of the additional shocking benefits of taking this simple vitamin:

1.  Activated vitamin D in the adrenal gland regulates tyrosine hydroxylase, the rate-limiting enzyme necessary for the production of dopamine, epinephrine, and norepinephrine.

2.  Low vitamin D may contribute to chronic fatigue and depression. Seasonal affective disorder has been treated successfully with vitamin D. In a recent study covering 30 days of treatment, comparing vitamin D and two-hour daily use of "light boxes" (devices that emit a full spectrum light that simulates sunlight), depression completely resolved in the vitamin D group, but not in the light box group.

3.  Scientific journal *Clinical Rheumatology* reported that those suffering from vitamin D deficiency scored much higher on anxiety and depression tests than those who had healthy vitamin D levels.

4.  Infertility is associated with low vitamin D, and PMS has been completely reversed with the addition of calcium, magnesium, and vitamin D.

5.  Thousands of studies are showing that Vitamin D can lower your chances of certain cancers by 70%.

6.  Autoimmune disease, such as multiple sclerosis, Sjogren's syndrome, rheumatoid arthritis, thyroiditis, and Crohn's disease, has been linked with low vitamin D levels.

7. Vitamin D deficiency has been clearly linked with syndrome X. Syndrome X refers specifically to a group of health problems that can include insulin resistance (the inability to properly deal with dietary carbohydrates and sugars), abnormal blood fats (such as elevated cholesterol and triglycerides), being overweight, and high blood pressure.

8. Vitamin D is extremely effective at halting influenza infections. Flu vaccines, according to the latest scientific evidence, achieve a 1% reduction in influenza symptoms. Vitamin D appears to be 800% more effective than vaccines at preventing influenza infections in children.

Even if vitamin D could save America billions of dollars in reduced health care costs (which it can), we don't hear it being advertised because drug companies can't patent vitamin D. It's readily available to everyone for a few pennies a day.

## Dosage and Tips

The best form of vitamin D is vitamin D3, the exact same type made in your body by sunlight. Most physicians recommend between 1000 IU and 1500 IU daily; however, one study found that depression during winter months was significantly reduced among study subjects who took a daily dose of 4000 IU for a period of one year.

- Children below age 5 should take 35 IU per pound (of their weight).

- Children aged 5–10 should take 1,000–2500 IU per day

> **HEALTH TIP: Always take vitamin D with a meal. Vitamin D is a fat-soluble vitamin and can only be absorbed when eaten with a fat. Do not take it late in the day because it increases serotonin and can cause sleep issues.**

# FISH OILS AND DHA

Little did Johanna Budwig know when she was studying omega-3 fatty acids that she was finding a groundbreaking cure for mental and childhood behavior disorders. Yes, in the 1950s, this German biochemist was reversing cancer and heart disease with omega-3 fatty acids. Later, scientists at Harvard picked up where Budwig's research stopped. They discovered the link between our brain health and omega-3 essential fatty acids. The conclusion was straightforward: a lack of essential fatty acids can contribute to mood imbalances, such as depression and bipolar disorder. Harvard researchers found that adding therapeutic doses of omega-3 into your diet can help eliminate these disorders.

DHA (docosahexaenoic acid) is found in fish oils. Scientists have found that DHA levels are low in alcoholics and in women right after giving birth. Apparently, alcohol depletes DHA levels. This causes a cycle of more alcohol and more depression.

Women in their postpartum period often get "the blues." Why is this so common? Well, babies need DHA for proper brain development, so in the last stages of pregnancy, the baby "pulls" DHA from the mother's stores. This is found to be the cause of postpartum depression. Adding DHA during your third trimester has been shown to help with the "baby blues," but even more interesting is that it can increase babies' IQ scores.

## Dosage and Tips

I recommend taking 1000 mg of omega-3 with breakfast, lunch, and dinner. Since the manufacturing of supplements like omega-3 fatty acids is not closely regulated, it is important to choose a trustworthy manufacturer. Look for the "USP" symbol; this means that the supplement has been tested and contains the right ingredients in the right amounts. Some omega-3 supplements derived from fish contain heavy metals and other toxins. Often, these supplements are purified in order to remove these toxins. Make sure to choose an omega-3 fatty acid supplement from a reputable manufacturer.

You may find that storing fish oil supplements in the freezer helps prevent some of the bothersome side effects of fish oil (such as a fishy aftertaste). This may also prevent fish oil supplements from becoming rancid. If you have any chronic health problems or take any prescription medications, you should check with your healthcare provider before taking omega-3 fatty acids.

## 5-HTP: Serotonin Booster

**Note:** *Do not take 5-HTP with a prescription antidepressant. Getting off antidepressants is tough; I have many clients transitioning right now. I would recommend getting a personal consultation on how to transition.*

Anxiety, depression, and obesity are issues I see everyday with clients, each issue reinforcing the other. Clients don't understand why they feel the way they do and want to "snap out of it." Our brain biochemistry plays a huge part in our moods, which can drive us to unhealthy eating behaviors. A nutritional supplement called 5-HTP (5-hydroxy-L-tryptophan) has been a miracle cure for my clients. According to scientist Michael Murray, N.D., "Numerous double-blind studies have shown 5-HTP to be as effective as antidepressant drugs, but it is better tolerated and is associated with fewer and much milder side effects. The body converts tryptophan, an amino acid (protein) found in food, into 5-HTP, which is used to make serotonin; an important brain chemical regulating mood, behavior, appetite, and sleep."

In Europe, 5-HTP has been used for decades as a standard treatment for depression, sleep problems, weight loss, and other medical problems. It is now starting to be used in the US. Scientific studies find that 5-HTP is a safe, natural way to increase the brain serotonin levels. Interestingly, 5-HTP has been found to produce results equal to or better than those of standard synthetic drugs used in the problems arising from serotonin deficiency or depression. Dr. Ray Sahelian, M.D., author of *5-HTP: Nature's Serotonin Solution*, believes 5-HTP holds a great deal of promise. He states, "5-HTP helps control appetite, improve[s] mood, and reduce[s] anxiety." Sounds good to me — sign me up!

## How Does 5-HTP Work?

After adding in amino acids to their diets, patients typically have positive results in three to four weeks, but in acute cases, there is often a significant improvement in a matter of days. Many of my clients are on powerful drugs called psychotropics, which include Valium and Prozac, to control their anxiety or depression. My goal is to increase my patient's amino acid reserves so they can eventually discontinue these drugs. However, this is not always possible or advisable in all cases, so the goal then becomes reducing the potential toxicity of the psychotropics, which will often reduce the side effects. It all comes down to brain chemicals. When people take Prozac for depression, they're actually trying to biochemically elevate their serotonin levels. When people take Valium and the other benzodiazepine drugs for anxiety, they're trying to elevate their GABA levels. People with deficiencies in serotonin tend to be depressed, while people without enough GABA suffer anxiety. What I do is substitute the natural neurotransmitters or their amino acid precursors for the psychotropic drugs. The result is more thorough healing with no side effects.

> **FAT BURNING TIP: The Irony of Antidepressants**
>
> Weight gain is a common side effect of many antidepressants and mood stabilizer medications. All antidepressants have the potential to cause weight gain; most people are unaware that weight gain is one of the most common side effects associated with Zoloft, Paxil, Prozac, Zyprexa, and many other behavioral drugs until it is too late. Ironically, this common side effect causes an increase in depression as it can seriously impact self-esteem. Many prescription drugs cause the liver to be tired and toxic. A toxic liver causes low moods and inability to burn fat efficiently. 5-HTP is a natural antidepressant that can actually help decrease cravings to assist in weight loss.

The first step in reversing anxiety and depression is to see which factors are at play. For example, there may be a genetic factor involved in which a person is somewhat predisposed at birth to be lacking in a specific neurotransmitter. Inadequate diet and nutrition is another factor that can leave one's system deficient in key minerals. The stress of today's fast-paced lifestyle may also deplete the body's reserves of amino acids and vital nutrients. One client had an undiagnosed toxic response to baked potatoes, which she ate every day thinking they were good for her. Some people have brain allergies to foods they eat regularly. These can show up like depression, when the cause is actually a chronic food allergy response.

Natural ways to correct the biochemical pathways associated with anxiety and depression are by elevating levels of key nutrients called amino acids, which are precursors to the neurotransmitters. The body does the rest on its own. In most cases, about 50% of people require an ongoing maintenance level of amino acids to keep their anxiety or depression under control, while others are able to eventually discontinue these supplements.

Somehow, the use of amino acids rather than pharmaceutical medicine seems to empower and even motivate people to get well. People who take nutrients under proper guidance seem to have a sense of power over what's happening to them, whereas many people taking pharmaceutical medications often feel that they're surrendering to some mystery, a feeling that is quite upsetting.

Mood and sleep disorders are imbalances in monoamine neurotransmitters. Having low levels of serotonin is an acknowledged factor in depression, obesity, and anxiety. Serotonin is a monoamine compound, chemically related to amino acid derivatives such as 5-HTP. Serotonin also increases levels of endorphins and many other neurotransmitters, which help decrease our recurrence of depression and low moods.

When levels of serotonin fall, your body senses starvation. To protect itself, your body starts to crave carbohydrates. Serotonin levels fall after you go too long without eating, and that encourages your body to start filling itself. People who use 5-HTP to keep their serotonin level up have more positive experience when dieting. Dr. Oz's book *YOU: On a Diet* had a six-week study of 5-HTP and dieters. The group of dieters using 5-HTP lost an average of 12 pounds, while the control group lost an average of four. Ninety percent of women taking at least 300 mg of 5-HTP report satiety while on a diet.

## 5-HTP and Depression

Pharmaceutical antidepressants, like Prozac, Zoloft and Paxil, work by blocking the deprivation of serotonin after it has performed its job, to bridge the gaps between nerve cells. These drugs, called SSRIs (selective serotonin re-uptake inhibitors) produce considerable unpleasant side effects, and do not work effectively unless the body is producing sufficient levels of serotonin in the first place. Vegetarians are often lacking enough amino acids to produce serotonin.

There have been controlled scientific studies comparing 5-HTP to SSRI drugs, specifically the drug fluvoxamine, also known as Luvox, and the drug Prozac. Participants receiving 5-HTP were found to have experienced a slightly better and faster relief than those who were given fluvoxamine, and a larger percentage of them had a positive reaction to 5-HTP. One study found that even though their serotonin levels increased, one in five participants who responded positively to 5-HTP relapses after one month because levels of other brain chemicals, known as monoamines, decreased. These patients responded terrifically to additional supplementation with the amino acid tyrosine. I use a product that has both 200 mg of 5-HTP and 100 mg of L-tyrosine for clients.

## 5-HTP and Obesity

Three clinical studies using a placebo and 5-HTP established that 5-HTP can be successful in assisting weight loss in overweight patients. It helps by creating feelings of satiety. People taking 5-HTP lost three to five times more weight as those who were taking a placebo.

## 5-HTP and Insomnia

5- HTP provides the fastest, most effective, and most unfailing results in treating insomnia. It is an effective alternative for people suffering with sleep issues. It is a safe and natural supplement compared to prescription and over-the-counter sleep medicines. Prescription sleep medications slow metabolism. 5-HTP improves the quality of sleep; most over-the-counter and pharmaceutical medications will knock you out, but don't increase REM sleep, which is the quality sleep we are looking for. 5-HTP lengthens REM sleep by about 25 percent, while at the same time lengthening deep sleep stages 3 and 4 without increasing total sleep time. 5-HTP accomplishes this by shortening the amount of time you spend in sleep stages 1 and 2, which are the least important stages of sleep. The higher the dose, the more time spent in REM. By shifting the balance of the sleep cycle, 5-HTP makes sleep more restful and rejuvenating. Instead of waking up feeling just as tired and "hung-over" as many people feel with medications like Tylenol PM, people taking 5- HTP feel energetic and well rested. When we get quality sleep, we dream more efficiently and wake up with our physical and mental batteries fully charged. The effectiveness of 5-HTP on sleep stages is dose-related; taking higher doses generates a greater impact, but usually a lower dose is sufficient. Higher doses may create more dreams or nightmares due to abnormally long REM sleep.

## 5-HTP and Headaches

Scientific studies find that 5-HTP is as successful as pharmaceutical drugs in decreasing symptoms of migraine headaches, because of the increase in serotonin.

## Dosage Recommendations
* 200–400 mg per night
* Always check with your doctor before starting a supplement regimen.

- The following is a testimonial from a client healing herself through proper nutrition:

*Dear Maria,*

*I can't thank you enough for all the things you've done. You are doing an incredible job! So please keep doing it! You make a difference, you really make this world a better place — thank you, thank you, thank you!*

*My journey on "your way" started in August, after my second miscarriage; I was suffering from nausea, indigestion, diarrhea, acid reflux, burning pain in my abdomen, hemorrhoids, joint and muscle pain, acne, hair loss and what not — you know, all the possible side effects of high dose antibiotics, antifungal and other prescribed post-surgical treatments. I was desperate for answers and the answer came from a dear friend of mine with an invitation to your [Facebook] group. The first thing I read there was something about gluten. I suddenly remembered that an endocrinologist had mentioned something like that a couple years before, when I'd been planning my first pregnancy — which wasn't a success either. However, at that time, all I knew about gluten intolerance was that it gives you some GI tract discomfort and I figured, oh well, almost everyone else has it and don't do a thing about it. Thus, having read a great amount of gluten intolerance facts from your blog, first of all I decided to eliminate all the gluten from my everyday meals. And by the way, that oat-meal all doctors like to prescribe with the heavy treatment (to ease the liver damage) gave me the most awful acid reflux, even after a single teaspoon, even without sugar. The only thing that would be actually soothing was something no sane doctor would suggest — lard and thick broth (which I also discovered in your blog and it gave me some confirmation on what I was doing)!*

*Then I came to the conclusion to eliminate all the rest of the bad stuff. You should've seen my husband begging me not to throw his candies and cookies away, just like a little boy! Since we don't have those sweeteners you write about here in Russia, we've excluded all the treats, even the "healthified" ones. In just a week of this strict diet we stopped thinking about anything sweet, not even fruit; we simply didn't need those anymore! In just a week, most of my* symptoms either disappeared or started fading away. Besides, my husband's apron—that's what I call his wheat belly—started melting away and so did his complaints. As for myself, I'm not a scale person, I believe in good old jeans (jeans don't lie) and as long as I could fit myself into size 4 I was happy. But I haven't been that happy lately, to be honest. Well, I became a size 1 in just two weeks! We've been this way for about 5 weeks now, and even though we never dine before 10 p.m.—and it's a solid meal, not just some kind of a snack—we keep losing our weight.

Now that we don't have cravings, it's absolutely effortless! My husband's joints feel fine now after years of pain! My body has never been so responsive and flexible, and here, believe me, I know what I'm talking about since I'm a yoga teacher. And that's another paradox. Food is always a very sensitive question for yoga followers; on one hand, flash eating is wrong, but on the other, we're not in India; the climate, the environment, and even the bodies differ! I knew that the real yoga diet doesn't fit most people. I could torture myself as long as I was willing to, but I knew that eating nuts and grapefruit for months is not a healthy way and it was the only way for me to maintain my look and to feel tolerable. But that was my choice and I could not suggest that to my clients for it's wrong. So whenever someone asked me to give some recommendations on eating, I'd just describe the Ayurvedic way, or the traditional "healthy" way, with cereal and skim milk for breakfast or a sport protein fat-free diet, neither of which were good for myself.

The only time I was feeling fine about the meals was when I was on Prozac, but that's just because you don't care whether you eat or not at all! And this year, after my second miscarriage—which, in fact, could also have happened because of gluten intolerance—I was sure I would end up taking Prozac again. I was too weak for exercise to handle my despair and devastation, ready to make the lives of everyone around myself just as miserable. And here I am, getting calmer, fitter, happier day by day.

I realize I'm not completely there yet, but it's a great start. Starting from this coming weekend I quit cheating (no more wine whatsoever); I was too tired *of those mood swings and skin problems afterwards, that cheating didn't seem like fun anymore. I'm taking all the supportive things [like supplements] you wrote about and am healing. I translate your articles just so my family members and friends who don't understand English can also get this vital information! Thank you for being there for us, helping and nurturing every single day! I can go on and on describing all the unbelievable things that have been happening to us since we've started it your way, but like I said, I can't thank you enough!*

*—Irina*

*(P.S. This [note] is from Russia!)*

## GLUTAMINE: GABA BOOSTER

Glutamine is very therapeutic for our digestive system; remember, our moods come from our gut. Intestinal health is important because it is the transport of fuel and nutrients. In this case, glutamine is the fuel that nourishes the cells that line the digestive track and intestines. Time and time again, studies have shown that a therapeutic dose of supplemental glutamine protects against aspirin-induced gastric lesions and helps heal painful ulcers. In fact, an old folk remedy for ulcers is cabbage juice, which is very high in glutamine. Stomach problems, such as colitis and Crohn's disease, can be calmed by glutamine. Glutamine can be used whenever there are any stomach problems, from something as simple as drinking too much alcohol (alcoholic-induced gastritis) to ulcers, diarrhea, or even more serious problems such as inflammatory bowel disease.

Glutamine is also beneficial for a variety of other health issues. The following points detail some benefits of glutamine:

1.  Glutamine can help prevent both depression and fatigue and can also help us create neurotransmitters in the brain, which help relax us while elevating our mood. In the brain, glutamine is transformed to glutamic acid and boosts the amount of GABA (gamma-aminobutyric acid) in our bodies. Both glutamic acid and GABA are considered "brain fuel" because they are necessary for everyday mental function.

2. Glutamine reduces cravings for high-glycemic carbohydrates and can make your weight loss plan a lot easier.

3. Many studies have found that therapeutic amounts of glutamine help prevent the harmful effects of alcohol on the brain and may also decrease alcohol (as well as sugar) cravings.

4. Glutamine is essential to our immune system because it is utilized by white blood cells. Glutamine is now used in some hospitals intravenously to speed up recovery of patients. The better you develop your muscles through exercise, the more glutamine they will produce, which is one of the reasons fit people get sick less often.

## Dosage Recommendation

A recent study published by *The American Journal of Clinical Nutrition* has shown that oral supplementation with as little as 2 grams of glutamine significantly enhanced patients' overall health.

Glutamine is a safe substance found in protein. Dosages of up to 21 grams a day have been demonstrated to have no negative side effects. High glutamine levels also support brain function, including better alertness. Taking 2 mg before bed increases human growth hormone. I recommend 3 grams three times a day on an empty stomach to heal the gut and increase GABA.

## PHENYLALANINE AND L-TYROSINE: DOPAMINE BOOSTER

Phenylalanine is an essential amino acid (meaning it cannot be produced by the body) and thus must be obtained through the diet. Phenylalanine is used in different biochemical processes to produce neurotransmitters, dopamine, norepinephrine, and epinephrine. The body converts phenylalanine into tyrosine, another amino acid essential for making proteins, thyroid hormones, and the brain chemicals dopamine and norepinephrine. Symptoms of phenylalanine deficiency include confusion, lack of energy, decreased alertness, decreased memory, and diminished appetite. Supplementation with both tyrosine and phenylalanine leads to alertness and mental arousal.

Phenylalanine and tyrosine are sometimes prescribed as antidepressants. I recommend these amino acids for appetite control as well. Phenylalanine helps trigger the release of an appetite-suppressing hormone in the gut called cholecystokinin. Most individuals who take either of these amino acids notice improved alertness, arousal, and mood, and notice a small loss in appetite.

I have numerous clients who start taking these amino acids who want to have a "caffeine" boost in the morning without the coffee. Tyrosine side effects can occur on high doses, which limits the usefulness of this amino acid.

Phenylalanine is available in the following three forms: L-phenylalanine, the natural form of phenylalanine found in proteins throughout the body; D-phenylalanine, a mirror image of L-phenylalanine that is synthesized in a laboratory; and DL-phenylalanine, a combination of the previous two forms.

The D form of phenylalanine is used to decrease pain. The L form is used as a mood enhancer, stimulant, and appetite suppressant. DL-phenylalanine is used by the brain to make norepinephrine, which is our brains' version of adrenaline. Adrenaline is a neurotransmitter depleted by stress, caffeine, exercise addiction, pollution, nicotine, and many pharmacological and recreational drugs. DL-phenylalanine also helps replace dopamine, the neurotransmitter responsible for feelings connected with self-confidence, sexual pleasure, and euphoria.

## TYROSINE

Tyrosine is a nonessential amino acid synthesized in the body from phenylalanine. It is an important factor for biosynthesis of the brain neurotransmitters epinephrine, norepinephrine, and dopamine. Tyrosine is also used to produce one of the major hormones, thyroxine, which plays an important role in controlling metabolic rate, skin health, mental health, and growth rate. Tyrosine is defined as the following:

- A precursor for biosynthesis of neurotransmitters
- A precursor for adrenaline and thyroid hormones
- Used to treat depression, anxiety, and allergies
- Combined with tryptophan to treat drug abuse
- An appetite suppressor
- Tyrosine deficiency will result in depression and mood disorders
- As a dietary precursor, it is one of the major nutritional ingredients that affects neurotransmitter synthesis and brain functions

Tyrosine is specifically used to treat depression because it is a precursor for those neurotransmitters that are responsible for transmitting nerve impulses and that are essential for preventing depression. Tyrosine has been tested on humans for increasing their endurance of anxiety and stress under fatigue. It has been proven in research studies that tyrosine supplementation results in increased performance.

Below are some of the benefits of supplementing with phenylalanine and tyrosine.

1. Phenylalanine may be effective in decreasing chronic pain, hunger, and depressed feelings.

2. L-tyrosine shares some of the characteristics of phenylalanine and may be effective in decreasing symptoms of Parkinson's disease and certain thyroid disorders.

3. The group of neurotrophin proteins, including nerve growth factor, brain-derived nerve factor, and neurotrophins (NT-3, NT-4/5, and 6), requires tyrosine and tryptophan as precursors to synthesis.

4. Dietary precursors, such as phenylalanine, tyrosine, tryptophan, and choline, promote the formation of neurotransmitters in the brain.

Tyrosine does all of the above except for one thing; it does not decrease chocolate cravings that are connected to beta phenylethylamine, a neuro-modulator associated with mood enhancement and sexual stimulation.

Tyrosine does not appear to be as active in this craving as DL-phenylala-nine. This is the reason some people refer to chocolate as a sexual stimulant. Unfortunately, all the extra sugar from consuming the amount of chocolate needed for sexual stimulation would also stimulate weight gain. If you are a chocoholic and want to lower your intake, phenylalanine can help a lot. Cravings are not a lack of willpower, they are truly a chemical imbalance!

## Weight Loss

Many ex-smokers gain weight after they quit smoking and use weight gain as a reason to not stop. Phenylalanine encourages the hypothalamus in the brain to release CCK (cholecystokinin), the hormone responsible for signaling fullness. Using phenylalanine helps eliminate the weight gain excuse.

One important thing to note is that DL-phenylalanine is not the same as phenylpropanolamine (a form of amphetamine). Phenylpropanolamine is an appetite suppressant used in several over-the-counter diet pills. These are harmful because they cause the brain to use up its stores of norepinephrine without stimulating it to produce more. On average, dieters stops taking the diet pill after about two weeks, which consequently causes "the blues" and low energy since they have little to no norepinephrine. These dieters then gorge on food and end up gaining more weight than before.

## Smoking and Drug Addiction

Why is it so hard to quit? There is evidence to support the idea that smoking releases dopamine into the brain. As a result, smokers get a rise in dopamine by "lighting-up." Quitting becomes much easier with therapeutic doses of phenylalanine.

Studies also show that cocaine users who are trying to quit have higher success when supplementing with DL-phenylalanine, L-theanine and L-glutamine. The chronic use of cocaine ultimately depletes dopamine and norepinephrine from the brain without replacing the key neurotransmitters. As dopamine is created from precursors such as DL-phenylalanine and theanine, dopamine reserves are rebuilt, finally overcoming the dopamine depletion. The use of DL-phenylalanine on a regular basis may be a cure for those who are trying to quit. One of cocaine's and other recreational drugs' main effects is the blocking of the reuptake of dopamine in the brain; this results in an increase in dopamine levels associated with the euphoric trait of the drug. However, constant use of drugs can lead to too much dopamine reduction and recovery is difficult.

In addition, drug use also causes various nutritional deficiencies. It is important to increase intake of certain vitamins and minerals, particularly vitamin C, pantothenic acid (vitamin B5), pyridoxal phosphate (B6), magnesium, and zinc. Vitamins B6 and C are important co-factors in the synthesis structure of dopamine, serotonin, and GABA.

## Dosage and Precautions

Phenylalanine and tyrosine should be used with caution by those with hypertension, phenylketonuria (PKU) (a rare genetic defect of the brain), or a preexisting pigmented melanoma. They also should not be used in combination with antidepressant drugs. Persons who have PKU cannot process phenylalanine. (This includes those born with a genetic deficiency that prevents them from metabolizing phenylalanine.) There have been reports that L-phenylalanine can promote high blood pressure in those predisposed to hypertension. Therefore, it is important to start off using smaller doses of phenylalanine, about 500 mg a day, and slowly work up to 1500 mg a day. Monitoring the first few months on phenylalanine can help detect blood pressure increases in the minority of people who will have this symptom.

DL-phenylalanine competes with other amino acids. It has to be able to pass through the stomach and blood-brain barrier without competition. Take phenylalanine on an empty stomach 15 to 20 minutes before eating. Avoid taking it with other amino acids. It is recommended to start with 500–1,000 mg as soon as you awake. Some people take another 500–1,000 mg four to six hours later for that extra "lift." Taking it too close to bedtime may keep you awake. Some people build up (after taking lower doses for a couple of weeks) to 2,000 mg in the morning and 2,000 mg in the evening.

There has to be significant amounts of vitamin B6 and vitamin C present in your bloodstream in order for phenylalanine (or tyrosine) to work. Taking 50–200 mg of Vitamin B6 and 3,000–4,000 mg of vitamin C divided throughout the day does a great job. Over time, healthy levels of norepinephrine are depleted by caffeine and other factors mentioned above if it is not replaced. Phenylalanine does an awesome job replacing this key neurotransmitter.

## MORE ON MAGNESIUM

What mineral is needed by every cell in the body, yet odds are you don't get enough of it? Hint: It's not calcium. Give up? It's magnesium. It gets little attention now, but rising evidence suggests that magnesium benefits your heart and bones, plus it may help prevent diabetes and migraine headaches. Magnesium is the fourth most abundant mineral in the body and is vital to a healthy body. Roughly 50% of total body magnesium is found in bone. The other half is found inside the cells of body tissues and organs. The symptoms of a magnesium deficiency include anxiety, depression, restlessness, confusion, irritability, brain fog, fatigue, irregular heartbeat, and tight, aching muscles.

In a magnesium deficiency, neuronal requirements for magnesium may not be met and may be causing neuronal damage, which manifests as depression. A therapeutic dose of magnesium is found to be effective in treating depression resulting from intra-neuronal magnesium deficits. The magnesium ion neuronal deficits can be induced by stress hormones, excessive dietary calcium, as well as dietary deficiencies of magnesium. Studies show rapid recovery (less than a week) from depression using 300 mg of quality magnesium with each meal and at bedtime.

Dietary deficiencies of magnesium, coupled with excess calcium and stress, may cause many cases of other related symptoms, including agitation, anxiety, irritability, confusion, asthenia, sleeplessness, headache, delirium, hallucinations, and hyperexcitability, with each of these having been studied and documented.

Magnesium is essential for more than three hundred biochemical actions in the body. It is vital for healthy aging and disease prevention. Studies have shown that magnesium deficiencies correlate to Alzheimer's and Parkinson's. Deficiencies also cause muscle spasms, pain, insomnia, and fatigue. Magnesium assists in maintaining muscle mass, nerve function, a regular heart beat, it helps our immune system, and it keeps bones strong. Diabetics benefit from magnesium as it helps regulate blood sugar levels. In addition, it normalizes blood pressure and is known to be involved in energy metabolism and protein synthesis. There has been a lot of medical interest in using magnesium to avoid and manage disorders, such as cardiovascular disease, diabetes, and hypertension.

The health of our digestive system and the kidneys is jeopardized if we are deficient in magnesium. This mineral is absorbed in the intestines and then transported through the blood into the cells and tissues. Gastrointestinal disorders, such as Crohn's disease or a food allergy, can limit the body's ability to absorb magnesium. These disorders can deplete the body's stores of magnesium, and in extreme cases, may result in a magnesium deficiency. Chronic vomiting and diarrhea will also deplete magnesium levels. Alcohol abuse and uncontrolled diabetes are other causes of magnesium deficiency.

> **HEALTH TIP:** Do you have a "twitchy" eye? That's a common sign of a magnesium deficiency. Do not buy magnesium oxide to fix this problem. It won't help it and will most likely cause you to run to the nearest bathroom.

Early signs of magnesium deficiency include nausea, fatigue, or weakness. As magnesium deficiency gets worse, restless leg syndrome, numbness, muscle cramps, seizures, mood changes, and irregular heartbeats can occur. A severe magnesium deficiency can also deplete the levels of calcium in the blood. Americans have the highest dietary intake of calcium in the world, yet we have the highest rate of hip fractures. Hmmm … could a magnesium deficiency be the cause? Magnesium deficiency is also associated with low levels of potassium in the blood.

Magnesium is also being researched as a natural way to curb food cravings. It is found that as magnesium deficiencies increase, so do food cravings. Supplementing with a therapeutic dose of 600 mg of magnesium is a natural way to tame those unruly carbohydrate desires.

Adults as well as children should get at least 400 mg of magnesium a day. Are you getting enough? Three ounces of Halibut only provides 90 milligrams; one ounce of almonds provides 80 milligrams; and a cup of spinach is 75 milligrams. Eating a variety of nuts and dark-green leafy vegetables every day will help provide the recommended intakes of magnesium and will help maintain normal storage levels of this mineral. However, increasing magnesium through food may not be enough to restore extremely low magnesium levels to normal. Oral therapeutic doses of magnesium supplements in the form of magnesium citrate or magnesium glycinate is the best way to ensure proper levels.

## Health Benefits of Magnesium

- Aids in fighting depression
- Reduces food cravings
- Beneficial in the treatment of PMS
- Relieves restless leg syndrome
- Particularly important for maintaining a normal heart rhythm and is often used by physicians to treat irregular heartbeat or arrhythmia
- Beneficial for bladder problems in women, especially common disturbances in bladder control and the sense of "urgency"
- Helps in the treatment of high blood pressure
- Beneficial in the treatment of neuromuscular and nervous disorders
- Helps prevent kidney stones and gallstones
- Vital for a healthy immune system

- Keeps teeth healthy
- Used by the body to help maintain muscles, nerves, and bones.
- Increases energy metabolism and protein synthesis
- Helps regulate blood sugar levels
- Adequate intake of calcium, magnesium, and vitamin D coupled with overall proper nutrition and weight-bearing exercise throughout childhood and adulthood are the primary preventive measures for osteoporosis
- Useful in treatment of polio and post-polio syndrome
- Useful in the treatment of prostate problems
- Helps reduce stress

## Muscle building

Magnesium supplements are often times marketed as muscle enhancers and testosterone boosters. Magnesium is a natural muscle relaxant which is extremely helpful for rebuilding tired and overused muscles. If you are strength training, and I hope you are, then supplementing with magnesium before bed will help your muscles repair faster for the next day's feats. Athletes also run the risk of having a lower immune system because their bodies are more focused on their muscles, but adding magnesium can significantly boost their immune systems during times of serious exercise.

## Premenstrual Syndrome

Increasing evidence shows premenstrual syndrome might also be triggered by dietary deficiencies in certain vitamins or minerals, especially magnesium. A magnesium deficiency has a direct correlation to premenstrual syndrome. Magnesium levels in PMS patients have been shown to be significantly lower than in normal subjects. Many women with PMS have high sugar intakes, which lowers magnesium levels in the blood. Supplemental magnesium appears to be a great natural cure.

## Blood Pressure

Recent studies find that magnesium may play an important role in regulating blood pressure. The DASH study (Dietary Approaches to Stop Hypertension), a human clinical trial, suggested that high blood pressure could be significantly lowered by a diet high in magnesium, potassium, and calcium. Diets filled with fruits and vegetables, which are good sources of potassium and magnesium, are without fail linked to lower blood pressure.

A study examined the effect of various nutritional factors related to high blood pressure in over 30,000 US male health professionals. After four years, it was found that a lower risk of hypertension was associated with increased amounts of magnesium, potassium, and dietary fiber. A six-year study of 8,000 patients who were initially free of hypertension, found that the risk of developing hypertension increases if a magnesium deficiency occurred.

## Diabetes

Diabetes is the result of an insufficient production or use of insulin. Insulin converts sugar and starches in our diet into energy. Magnesium plays a significant function in carbohydrate metabolism by assisting the release and activity of insulin. A magnesium deficiency aggravates insulin resistance, a condition that starts the ball rolling for diabetes; deficiencies are commonly found in patients with type 2 diabetes. Kidneys possibly lose their ability to maintain magnesium levels during periods of elevated levels of blood glucose. Magnesium is lost due to the increase in urination. Supplementing with a therapeutic dose of magnesium may improve insulin levels.

## Cardiovascular Disease

Magnesium influences metabolism, diabetes, and high blood pressure, all of which increases the probability that magnesium influences cardiovascular disease. Extended surveys have connected higher blood levels of magnesium with a lower risk of heart disease. Some dietary surveys also found that higher magnesium levels may reduce the risk of having a stroke. Evidence also proves that low levels of magnesium increase the risk of abnormal heart rhythms, which adds to the risk of complications after a heart attack.

Researchers studied the effects of magnesium supplementation and the ability to walk on a treadmill, chest pain caused by exercise, and quality of life. Patients received either a therapeutic dose of 400 mg of magnesium citrate twice daily for six months or a placebo. At the end of the study period, researchers found that magnesium therapy significantly improved magnesium levels. Patients receiving magnesium had a 14 percent improvement in exercise duration and experienced less chest pain caused by exercise as compared to no change in the placebo group.

## Recommended Dose of Magnesium

Dietary magnesium does not pose a health risk, however therapeutic doses of magnesium in supplements can have unfavorable effects such as diarrhea. Choosing the correct form of magnesium will help prevent this undesired effect. Magnesium oxide is found in Milk of Magnesia, so of course that version of magnesium will cause diarrhea. Choose magnesium citrate or magnesium glycinate; these are highly absorbable forms and cannot be found in your typical retail store. Talk to your local health food store, nutritionist, or chiropractor. These versions are a little more expensive, but you are ensuring absorption of the nutrient — it is money well spent.

I recommend taking 400–800 mg of magnesium around 30 minutes before going to bed. Someone suffering from a medical condition or on medication that depletes magnesium may require more: up to 1,000 mg per day. Magnesium is a natural muscle relaxant that improves sleep. In addition to supplements, taking baths with magnesium salts provides added benefits. Absorbing magnesium through the skin stimulates the production of DHEA, the anti-aging hormone.

# WHAT NOW?

Follow these steps:

1. Eat lots of healthy fats. Our brain and cells are over 60% fat. Let's fuel our brain and cells with a well-formulated keto-adapted diet.

2. Eliminate all vegetable oils. Change your diet to restore fatty acid balance.

3. Add fresh organic herbs and spices to your cooking.

4. Decrease the amount of carbohydrates and sugar in your diet. High-carb diets cause high insulin levels, which cause your blood sugar to drop (what goes up must come down), and more cravings. Carbohydrates temporarily raise serotonin levels, but at a price.

5. Take antistress vitamins and minerals.

6. Go to bed on time and wake up at the same time each day. A lack of sleep strains your serotonin levels.

7. Reduce stress and simplify your life. It can be done.

8. Expose yourself to early morning sunlight or buy a specially designed light unit and use it each morning. Avoid bright light later in the day. Morning sunlight increases the level of melatonin in your bloodstream at night, which induces sleep and increases the level of serotonin.

9. Keep cool. Heat severely lowers serotonin levels because serotonin is used up in trying to cool down the body. People with low serotonin levels have trouble sweating and staying cool.

10. Exercise! Regular exercise increases both serotonin and dopamine and affects hormone systems as well. The role of exercise for both physical and mental health has been well recognized. Specifically, watching yourself lift weights and get stronger increases serotonin. Even if you are still overweight, watching your body be able to lift those weights lifts your moods.

11. Buy an air ionizer. I know it sounds weird, but air with negatively charged particles increases serotonin levels in the brain. Pollution eliminates naturally charged air in metropolitan areas. You can feel the

satisfying effects of negative ions wherever there is running water, like an ocean beach or a waterfall. The opposite (positive ions) are made by warm winds over dry land, which are known to increase violence and suicide. Crazy, but true!

# GOOD LUCK!

So with all of this information, I wish you luck in your journey to a healthy weight. I know this may all seem overwhelming and new, but try one new thing a week; maybe this week you will change your breakfast from cereal to eggs, next week start walking after dinner. 'Baby steps' are what worked for me. Instead of feeling overwhelmed, feel empowered by having the tools you need for a successful journey. No more deprivation diets of fat-free, man-made foods…real food, real satisfaction and a healthy brain.

# Notes

SELECTED REFERENCES

Belobrajdic DP, McIntosh GH, Owens JA. A high-whey-protein diet reduces body weight gain and alters insulin sensitivity relative to red meat in wistar rats. J Nutr. 2004 Jun;134(6):1454

Cangiano, C., et al. Eating behavior and adherence to dietary prescriptions in obese adult subjects treated with 5-hydroxytryptophan. American Journal of Clinical Nutrition. 1992 Nov;56(5):863-7.

Cappon JP, et al. Acute effects of high fat and high glucose meals on the growth hormone response to exercise. J Clin Endocrinol Metab. 1993 Jun;76(6):1418-22.

Clippinger, B., et al. Comparison of Meal Frequency and Macronutrient Composition on Changes in Total and Regional Body. Medicine & Science in Sports & Exercise 38(5 S): S69-S70, 2006.

Collier, S. R,, et al. Growth hormone responses to varying doses of oral arginine. Growth Hormone and IGF Research 15(2):136-139, 2005.

Dhiman, TR. "Conjugated Linoleic Acid Content of Milk from Cows Fed Different Diets" 1999 J Dairy Sci 82:2146-2156.

Hall, W. L., et al. Casein and whey exert different effects on plasma amino acid profiles, gastrointestinal hormone secretion and appetite. British Journal of Nutrition 89(2):239-248, 2003.

Hall WL, Millward DJ, Long SJ, Morgan LM. Casein and whey exert different effects on plasma amino acid profiles, gastrointestinal hormone secretion and appetite. Br Nutr. 2003 Feb;89(2):239-48.

Hayes, A. and Cribb, P. J. Effect of whey protein isolate on strength, body composition and muscle hypertrophy during resistance training. Curr Opin Clin Nutr Metab Care. 2008 Jan;11(1):40-4.

Markus CR, Olivier B, Panhuysen GE, et al. The bovine protein alpha-lactalbumin increases the plasma ratio of tryptophan to the other large neutral amino acids, and in vulnerable subjects raises brain serotonin activity, reduces cortisol concentration, and improves mood under stress. Am J Clin Nutr. 2000 Jun;71(6):1536-44.

Meeking DR, Wallace JD, Cuneo RC, Forsling M, Russell-Jones DL. Exercise-induced GH secretion is enhanced by the oral ingestion of melatonin in healthy adult male subjects. Eur J Endocrinol. Jul 1999;141(1):22-26.

Mercola J. Sweet Deception, Thomas Nelson, Inc, 2006.

Patel, S. R., et al. Association between Reduced Sleep and Weight Gain in Women. American Journal of Epidemiology 2006 164(10):947-954.

Powers ME, Yarrow JF, McCoy SC, Borst SE. Growth hormone isoform responses to GABA ingestion at rest and after exercise. Med Sci Sports Exerc. Jan 2008;40(1):104-110.

Spiegel, K., et al. Brief communication: Sleep curtailment in healthy young men is associated with decreased leptin levels, elevated ghrelin levels, and increased hunger and appetite. Ann Intern Med. 2004 Dec 7;141(11):846-50.

Swithers, S.E., et al. "A Role for Sweet Taste: Calorie Predictive Relations in Energy Regulation by Rats." Behavioral Neuroscience 2008, Vol. 122, No. 1, 161-173

Taheri S, Lin L, Austin D, Young T, Mignot E (2004) Short Sleep Duration Is Associated with Reduced Leptin, Elevated Ghrelin, and Increased Body Mass Index. PLoS Med 1(3): e62.

Supplemental choline has even shown promise in treating Alzheimer's Disease. (Today's Living, February, 1982)

Docosahexaenoic acid and omega-3 fatty acids in depression by Mischoulon D, Fava M Depression Clinical and Research Program, Department of Psychiatry, Massachusetts General Hospital and Harvard Medical School, Boston, Massachusetts, USA. Psychiatr Clin North Am 2000 Dec; 23(4):785-94; http://www.biopsychiatry.com/dhaomega.htm]

Omega-3 polyunsaturated fatty acid levels in the diet and in red blood cell membranes of depressed patients by Edwards R, Peet M, Shay J, Horrobin D University Department of Psychiatry, University of Sheffield, UK.J Affect Disord 1998 Mar; 48(2-3):149-55; http://www.biopsychiatry.com/omega3.html], [Omega 3 fatty acids in bipolar disorder: a preliminary double-blind, placebo-controlled trial by Stoll AL, Severus WE, Freeman MP, Rueter S, Zboyan HA, Diamond E, Cress KK, Marangell LB. Brigham and Women's Hospital, Department of Psychiatry, Harvard Medical School, Boston, Mass, USA. alstoll@mclean.harvard.edu Arch Gen Psychiatry 1999 May; 56(5):407-12; http://www.biopsychiatry.com/omega3.htm]

Essential fatty acids predict metabolites of serotonin and dopamine in cerebrospinal fluid among healthy control subjects, and early- and late-onset alcoholics by Hibbeln JR, Linnoila M, Umhau JC, Rawlings R, George DT, Salem N Jr Laboratory of Membrane Biochemistry and Biophysics, National Institute on Alcohol Abuse and Alcoholism, Bethesda, Maryland, USA. Biol Psychiatry 1998 Aug 15; 44(4):235-42; http://www.biopsychiatry.com/fattyacids.html]

Source: "Vitamin B Deficiencies" by Karen Railey; http://chetday.com/vitaminbdeficiencies.html